Atlas of Sleep Medicine

Atlas of Sleep Medicine

Lois E. Krahn, MD

Michael H. Silber, MBChB, FCP (SA)

Timothy I. Morgenthaler, MD

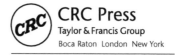

CRC Press
Taylor & Francis Group
Boca Raton London New York

CRC Press is an imprint of the
Taylor & Francis Group, an **informa** business

CRC Press
Taylor & Francis Group
6000 Broken Sound Parkway NW, Suite 300
Boca Raton, FL 33487-2742

First issued in paperback 2019

© 2011 by Taylor & Francis Group, LLC
CRC Press is an imprint of Taylor & Francis Group, an Informa business

No claim to original U.S. government works.

ISBN-13: 978-0-415-45008-9 (hbk)
ISBN-13: 978-0-367-38340-4 (pbk)

A CIP record for this book is available from the British Library.

Library of Congress Cataloging-in-Publication Data available on application.

Typeset by MPS Limited, a Macmillan Company

Visit the Taylor & Francis Web site at
http://www.taylorandfrancis.com

and the CRC Press Web site at
http://www.crcpress.com

Dedication

This book has been inspired by the patients who seek solutions and care from the Center for Sleep Medicine at Mayo Clinic.

Preface

This atlas is intended to provide an overview for the reader of the rich and ever-expanding field of sleep medicine. The authors, a multidisciplinary team of a psychiatrist, a neurologist, and a pulmonologist, have drawn upon multiple sources to illustrate the influence of both sleep and disordered sleep on the human condition. This volume touches upon several interdisciplinary topics, notably the history of sleep and sleep in animals, that exist on the periphery of the commonly accepted domain of medicine. Ideally, this atlas will inspire the reader to seek a greater understanding of the significance of sleep.

Lois E. Krahn, MD

Contents

Authors

Lois E. Krahn, MD Chair, Department of Psychiatry and Psychology and Consultant, Division of Pulmonary Medicine, Mayo Clinic, Scottsdale, Arizona; Professor of Psychiatry and Director for Education, College of Medicine, Mayo Clinic

Timothy I. Morgenthaler, MD Associate Chair for Quality, Department of Internal Medicine, and Consultant, Center for Sleep Medicine and Division of Pulmonary and Critical Care Medicine, Mayo Clinic, Rochester, Minnesota; Associate Professor of Medicine, College of Medicine, Mayo Clinic

Michael H. Silber, MBChB, FCP (SA) Co-Director, Center for Sleep Medicine and Consultant, Department of Neurology, Mayo Clinic, Rochester, Minnesota; Professor of Neurology, College of Medicine, Mayo Clinic

Contributor

Sarah Morgenthaler Bonnema, BA Department of Community and Family Health, University of South Florida, College of Public Health, Tampa, Florida

A History of Sleep and Sleep Medicine

Sarah Morgenthaler Bonnema, BA, and Timothy I. Morgenthaler, MD

ABBREVIATIONS

EEG, electroencephalograph; electroencephalographic

NREM, non–rapid eye movement

OSA, obstructive sleep apnea

REM, rapid eye movement

But this I very well know, that while I am asleep, I feel neither hope nor despair; I am free from pain and insensible of glory. Now blessings light on him that first invented this same sleep: it covers a man all over, thoughts and all, like a cloak; it is meat for the hungry, drink for the thirsty, heat for the cold, and cold for the hot. It is the current coin that purchases all the pleasures of the world cheap; and the balance that sets the king and the shepherd, the fool and the wise man even. There is only one thing, which somebody once put into my head, that I dislike in sleep; it is, that it resembles death; there is very little difference between a man in his first sleep, and a man in his last sleep.

(Sancho Panza speaking in *Don Quixote* by Miguel de Cervantes [Hertfordshire: Wordsworth Editions Limited, 1993. Part 2. Chapter 68. {Used with permission.}])

The medical specialty of sleep medicine has a brief history spanning only the past 25 to 50 years. Like other medical specialties, sleep medicine evolved in response to the increased prevalence and recognition of disease (in this case, sleep disorders) and to the availability of specialized methods to diagnose and treat them. Technological, economic, and sociological changes in the past century have outpaced our ability as organisms to adapt, ignoring our biological necessity for sleep quantity, quality, and timing. Arguably, the very factors that have increased our standard of living have contributed to an increased prevalence of sleep maladies. Artificial light has, in effect, shrunken the night, and 20% of the workforce in developing nations now works during the workers' circadian sleep period within the endogenous 24-hour internal sleep- and wake-related rhythm of humans (1). Mechanized transit enables the rapid traverse of multiple timelines, creating the chronobiological condition known as *jet lag*. Passive entertainment and work specialization have led to more sedentary pursuits. Coupled with the immense increase in food supply and our increasing consumption of processed foods, the sedentary lifestyle has resulted in an epidemic of obesity that contributes to obstructive sleep apnea (OSA) syndrome, one of the most common sleep disorders. Concurrent with these changes has been an explosion in the development of special-

ized knowledge about the biology of sleep and about measurement techniques to study sleep.

The history of sleep medicine may be new, but man's interest in sleep dates back to the earliest times. To examine it, we must consider not only science but also philosophy, art, law, and literature. History is dynamic. We can try to study and document what has gone before, but new learning often leads to a reinterpretation of the old such that our view of the past is not static. It is difficult to apply a satisfactory organization to a grand story spanning many centuries, but we have ambitiously organized this history into a survey of mankind's efforts to understand the purpose and nature of sleep, the experiences of sleep (including dreams and their meaning), the physiology of sleep, and the recognition and treatment of sleep disorders.

THE PURPOSE AND NATURE OF SLEEP

Sleep and Death, two twins of winged race,
Of matchless swiftness, but of silent pace.
(*The Iliad of Homer*, Book XVI [circa 850 BC]) (2)

Before the recent developments in sleep science, descriptions of sleep often took on two faces. On the one hand, sleep was viewed as a gift from the gods, as a welcome balm that restores energy and health, and as a sweet respite from the strife of life. On the other hand, sleep was identified with darkness, and thus at times was viewed as a consort of death and danger, as a vulnerable window into which the vilest evils might visit our unprotected souls. One of the oldest written references to sleep appears in the early chapters of Genesis in the Hebrew Bible (the Christian Old Testament) describing how Yahweh (God) placed Adam into a deep sleep, removed his rib, and created Eve (Figure 1; Table 1: Hebrew Words for Sleep) (3). An ancient Hindu text, *The Laws of Manu*, proposed that before the supreme being Svayambhu created the world, the universe "existed in the shape of Darkness, unperceived, destitute of distinctive marks, unattainable by reasoning, unknowable, wholly immersed, as it were, in deep sleep" (4).

From antiquity, sleep was seen as a time of inactivity and vulnerability to events that would be less likely to occur to a person while awake. Some fearsome warriors could be subdued only in their sleep, as was the case with the biblical hero Samson (Figure 2):

Having put him to sleep on her [Delilah's] lap, she called a man to shave off the seven braids of his hair, and so began to subdue him. And his strength left him (Judges 16:19 [NIV]) (5).

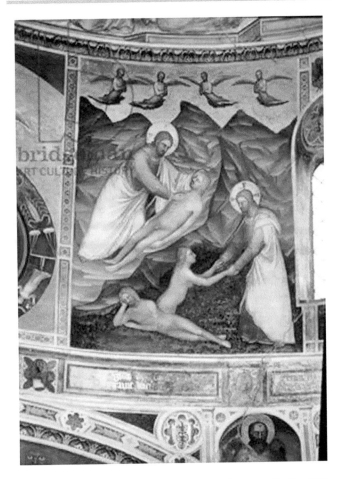

Figure 1 The Creation of Eve. In the Genesis account in the Bible, God causes an involuntary sleep to come over Adam (Hebrew word "Radum") that is sufficiently deep to allow the completion of the creation of Eve, apparently using Adam's rib as a template (upper panel of fresco). In the lower panel, Adam is depicted as sleeping on his right side during the act of creation. From early times onward, sleeping on the right side was advocated as a healthy posture, whereas supine sleeping was almost uniformly discouraged in ancient (and even in more contemporary) texts. (Baptistry fresco titled the *Creation of Man and Woman* by the Florentine painter Giusto dé Giovanni Menabuoi [circa 1320-1391].) (From the Basilica of St. Anthony in Padua, Italy.) (From Bridgeman Art Library International, New York, New York. [Used with permission.])

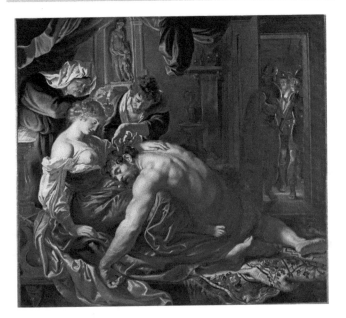

Figure 2 The Betrayal of Samson. Samson, the Jewish biblical hero endowed with supernatural strength, proved to have two weaknesses: his arrogance in believing himself invulnerable to the wiles of the Philistine woman Delilah, and the very real vulnerability of sleep. Here, after discovering from Samson that his uncut hair is the requisite for his strength, Delilah summons a servant to cut his hair while he sleeps. His waiting enemies, the Philistines (at the doorway) will then be able to easily subdue him (Judges 16:17-20). Throughout history and in literature and common experience, sleep has been seen as a compromising time. Historically, the sleeper has often been viewed as being more vulnerable to the action of supernatural forces that may influence dreams, and thus alter the understanding, attitudes, and actions of the victim. In literature the sleeper has been portrayed as being captured, killed, injured, or tricked. (Oil on wood painting titled *Samson and Delilah* [circa 1609-1610] by Peter Paul Rubens [1577-1640].) (From National Gallery, London/Art Resource, New York. [Used with permission.])

Table 1 Ancient Hebrew descriptors of different types of sleep[a]

Hebrew word	Context	Meaning (possible stage)
Tenumah	Isaiah 5:27 Psalm 76:6	Drowsy, lighter sleep (stage 1 sleep)
Yashen or shehah	Genesis 28:16 Genesis 31:40	Conscious thought that becomes unconscious and involuntary (stage 2)
Radam	Jonah 1:5-6 Genesis 2:21	Heavy or deep sleep (slow-wave sleep)
Tardemah	Genesis 15:12	Trancelike sleep, where thoughts continue to flow (REM sleep?)

Abbreviation: REM, rapid eye movement.
[a]Data from Ancoli-Israel S. "Sleep is not tangible" or what the Hebrew tradition has to say about sleep. Psychosom Med 2001; 63: 778-87.

In Homer's epic poem *The Odyssey* (6), Odysseus was powerless before the cannibalistic Cyclops Polyphemus while the Cyclops was awake, but he managed to engineer the escape of himself and his shipmates by maiming the single eye of the giant while he slept (Figure 3). The state of sleep seemed so vulnerable and still that the ancient Greeks believed that Hypnos, the god of sleep, and Thanatos, the god of death, were twin brothers and that sleep was a passive state barely differentiated from death (Figures 4 and 5). Millennia later, this view of sleep as being passive remained widely popular; in 1834 Robert Macnish wrote in his textbook *The Philosophy of Sleep* that sleep was a passive state on a continuum somewhere between wakefulness and death (7). Until the 1950s, this predominant view of sleep often served as a major impediment to sleep research, although luckily some historical figures looked past this misconception.

The Greek philosopher Plato (429-347 BC) was among the first scholars to speculate that sleep had an actual purpose other than as the rest near death; he postulated that its function was to cool the brain (8). His pupil Aristotle (384-322 BC) later refined this view, stating that one fell asleep as the result of a daily epileptic seizure, but that sleep then resided in and cooled

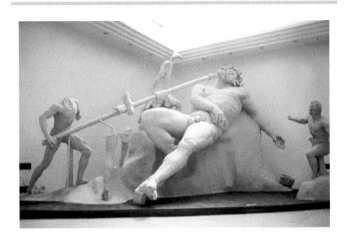

Figure 3 Blinding the Sleeping Cyclops. If sleep is a time of vulnerability, how much more so is the sleep following indulgence in strong drink! In the ancient legend told in Homer's *Odyssey*, the Cyclops Polyphemus dines on the ship's crew. To save themselves, they induce a deep (and defenseless) sleep in the Cyclops by giving him wine. Once the Cyclops is in this weakened condition, they are able to blind him by poking out his solitary eye. Afterward, they escape by clinging to the bellies of sheep that pass by the Cyclops when he allows them out of his cave to graze. (Statue in the Museo Archeologico Nazionale, Sperlonga, Italy.) (From Livius. [Used with permission.])

the heart, providing a time for food to digest (9). Aristotle believed that sleep facilitated rest, which was necessary for the conservation of life (10). For a time, alterations to Aristotle's views were minimal. The Greek physician Galen (circa AD 129-210) observed that "sleep and vigil" could benefit the person if applied correctly but could be harmful if applied incorrectly. The Islamic philosopher-scientist and Persian physician Avicenna (AD 973-1037) wrote that healthy persons must pay attention to their sleep because proper sleep is essential to the balance of the "humors." (Early Greek practitioners held that the wax and wane of four humors, identified as black bile, yellow bile, phlegm, and blood, determined one's health.)

Later reports in the scholarly literature emphasized the restorative imperative of sleep. In the sixteenth century, the Dutch physician Levinus Lemnius (1505-1568) described sleep as a period of revival:

> Sleepe is nothing else but a resting of the animall faculty, and a pawsing from the actions and businesse of the day, whereby the vertues of the body being faint, and the powers thereof being resolve, are revived and made fresh againe, and all the weary members and Senses recomforted (10).

In 1771 Johann August Unzer (1727-1799) wrote in his *Erste Gründe einer Physiologie der eigentlichen thierischen Natur thierischer Korper* (*Principles of a Physiology of the Proper Animal Nature of Animal Bodies*) that sleep was an instinctual reaction to the disagreeable sensation of fatigue (11). Eight years later the English physiologist George Henry Lewes commented that the function of sleep was to provide repose for the brain and senses in order to allow the nervous system to rest.

The struggle to understand the purpose of sleep continues to vex modern-day scientists and physicians. However, the most recent conceptualization of the sleeping patterns of both men and animals is that sleep is a way to conserve energy by keeping organisms inactive at inopportune times and active at required times. Sleep periods in certain species correlate with dietary availability; thus when food is not plentiful, activity is minimized. Sleep is also postulated to reverse changes in brain function caused by wakefulness such as neuronal oxidative stress, depletion of glycogen stores and neurogenesis-related proteins, and accumulation of neuronal adenosine (12).

DREAMING AND DREAMS

> *The minds of men, which with mighty movements bring forth mighty deeds, often in sleep do and dare just the same; they storm kings, are captured, join battle, raise a loud cry, as though being murdered—all without moving.*
> (Lucretius [98-55 BC]) (13)

Dream function and interpretation were by far the most dominant areas of sleep study in early history. Numerous accounts of prophetic dreams can be found in Judeo-Christian texts, Egyptian papyri, Sumerian inscriptions, and classic Greco-Roman literature (Figure 6). Interpretations of these dreams often served as turning points in history. Dreams allegedly guided the Roman emperor Julius Caesar (100-44 BC) in his decision to cross the Rubicon (14), the Carthaginian general Hannibal (circa 247-182 BC) in his decision to traverse the Alps, and the French philosopher René Descartes (1596-1650) in the development of his scientific methods, which included analytical geometry.

During the formative years of medicine, Greek physicians advocated that certain dreams had diagnostic properties. The first medical textbooks included dream interpretation manuals, indicating that "dreams were considered to be phenomena worthy of serious investigative inquiry" (15). One such textbook, *Regimen*, is a collection of medical treatises written sometime between 500 and 320 BC by a group of physicians known as the Hippocratic doctors (16). Its *Book IV: On Dreams* is particularly representative of these early roots of sleep medicine. The anonymous author of this text speculated that dreams were caused by the soul and contained either prophetic content useful for forecasting the future or diagnostic content that signified what ailed the body. The author had little confidence in the ability of physicians to interpret prophetic dreams but did encourage them to interpret diagnostic dreams. For example, he wrote that dreaming about mist, cloud, rain, or hail signified that the body was secreting extra phlegm. In 300 BC the Greek physician Herophilus (335-280 BC) introduced a slightly different dream classification method by suggesting that dreams fell into three categories: 1) those inspired or sent by a god, 2) "natural" dreams that the soul created to indicate what will come about, and 3) "compound" dreams that arise from a combination of our wishes and images of reality (17).

The great Greek medical scholars continued to develop their concepts of dreaming from these early theories. In the second century BC, the Greek diviner and author Artemidorus (18) wrote a dream interpretation manual titled the *Onirocriticon* (15). In this work he described six elements by which all dreams should be interpreted: law, occupation, names, time,

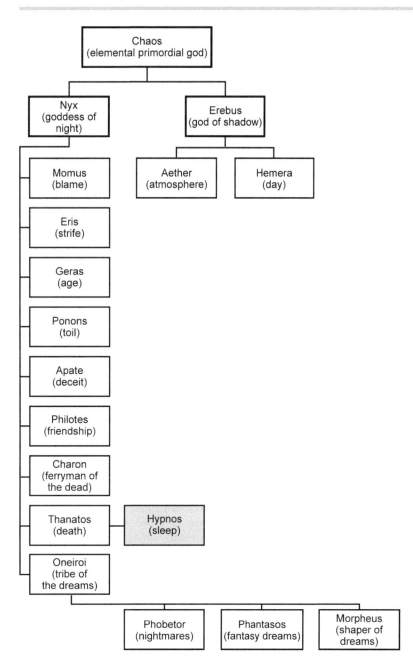

Figure 4 The Pedigree of Sleep in Greek Mythology. By some schemes, the progeny of Chaos are night (Nyx) and shadow (Erebus). The goddess Nyx, being one of the first-born primordial gods (Protogenoi), gives birth (often without any ascribed husband) to various aspects of the human condition, among them death (Thanatos) and sleep (Hypnos). Throughout much early history, death and sleep were depicted as being nearly alike; to the Greeks, they were like (twin) brothers of the same mother. The palace of Hypnos was portrayed as a dark cave where the sun never shone, and with poppies and other hypnogogic plants gracing its entrance. Images often show Hypnos bedecked with wings on his feet, shoulders, or brow (so he could rise into the sky in the train of mother Nyx), with his hands often holding either a horn of sleep-inducing opium, a poppy stem, or a branch of dripping water from the river Lethe (forgetfulness). He was also often paired with his brothers (or sons, depending on the source), the Oneroi (brothers of dreams). The ancient Greeks developed several schemas about the nature and meaning of dreams.

custom, and nature. Dreams in agreement with these elements indicated positive outcomes; those not in agreement foreshadowed negative outcomes.

Galen also studied dreams intently, and in his essay "On Diagnosis in Dreams," he wrote of a wrestler who in his dreams "seemed to be standing in a receptacle of blood" (19). Galen noted that it was later determined that this wrestler had an abundance of blood and needed to be purged. Galen explained that

> in sleep, the soul, having gone into the depths of the body and retreated from the external perceptions, perceives the dispositions throughout the body and forms an impression of all that it reaches out to. (19)

Nightmares were a popular topic, regardless of any sort of dream classification scheme (Figure 7). The ancient Greeks blamed nightmares on the gods, primarily the three sons (or brothers, according to some pedigrees [Figures 4 and 5]) of the Greek god of sleep, Hypnos (from which is derived the word *hypnosis*), who was the twin of Thanatos (*death*): 1) Phobetor (*phobia*), who appeared in dreams in the form of animals or monsters; 2) Morpheus (*morphine*), the god of dreams, who was responsible for the human elements of dreams; and 3) Phantasos (*phantasm*), who appeared in dreams in the form of inanimate objects. Their visits were the result of the sleeper's gluttony, epilepsy, fever, or other physical conditions.

In Roman times the attacking spirit in the nightmare was known as the *incubus,* an envoy from hell who raped women in

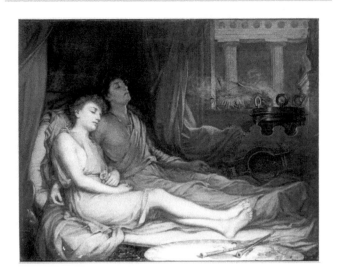

Figure 5 Hypnos and Thanatos. In Greek mythology, sleep (Hypnos, at left) and death (Thanatos, at right) are closely related, perhaps even twins. Note the poppies, from which were derived laudanum and opium for inducing sleep and dreamlike states. (Oil on canvas painting titled *Sleep and His Half-Brother Death* [1874] by the English pre-Raphaelite painter John William Waterhouse.) (From Fine Art Photographic Library, London/Art Resource, New York. [Used with permission.])

the question of where thoughts came from and entertained the possibility that dreams were ideas originating in the sleeping brain (22). The father of nine children, he was fascinated with how infants smile:

> A few days—sometimes a few hours—after they are born we see them smile in their sleep. But it's not easy to guess what they are smiling at, for it's not until some months later that they smile at anything while awake. It is also common to see them move their lips, as if they were sucking, while they are asleep.
>
> These things seem to reveal some working of the imagination (22).

These observed activities of sleep in infants may be the earliest written observation of what is called *active sleep* that would later be found to be the equivalent of rapid eye movement (REM) sleep. In 1896 Sarah Weed and Florence Hallam also recorded observations on the circadian nature of dreams. They noted that only "20 dreams (out of 150) were caused by external stimuli," and that dreams that occurred from 5 AM to 6:30 AM were "the most frequent, most interesting, most vivid and most varied" (13).

If dreams do not originate from external stimuli or demons or the gods, if they might be the seat of imagination or original thought, and if they are indeed embedded in the human experience, then what is their purpose? Some authors have suggested that dreams are a way for our "selves" to break through to thoughts that we could not otherwise identify. In 1811 the Scottish philosopher Dugald Stewart (1753-1823) suggested that we do not gain any new abilities or capacities in dreams; rather, dreams cause us to lose our ability to control our thoughts and wills (11). The American neurologist Edward H. Clarke wrote in 1878 that a dream is "the unconscious cerebration of that portion of the brain over which sleep has no power," the result of the brain acting on itself in sleep. The most famous dream theory to emerge from this time period, however, was that suggested by the Austrian physician and founder of psychoanalysis Sigmund Freud, who believed that dreams serve as a window onto the unconscious:

> The interpretation of dreams is the royal road to a knowledge of the unconscious activities of the mind (23).

Freud's landmark book, *The Interpretation of Dreams*, was published in 1899. The book sold an unimpressive 351 copies in its first six years in print yet went on to revolutionize the world of psychology and philosophy (23).

The discovery in the early 1950s by Eugene Aserinsky and Nathaniel Kleitman of REM sleep (that period of sleep when our most vivid dreams occur) as a distinct periodic physiological process different from non–rapid eye movement (NREM) sleep ushered in a whole new opportunity to study the phenomenon of dream sleep quantitatively, but it also introduced a new list of questions, speculations, and observations (Figure 9) (24). Although these later developments largely supplanted the dream interpretation methods of Freud, the precise function of REM remains incompletely understood.

THE MECHANICS OF SLEEP

And yet there is so much difference betwixt myself and myself, within that moment wherein I pass from waking to sleeping, or return from sleeping to waking!
(Saint Augustine of Hippo [circa AD 398]) (25)

their sleep (Figure 8). The fourth-century theologian Saint Augustine of Hippo (AD 354-430) wrote in his classic work, *The City of God* (20), that incubi "often made wicked assaults upon women, and satisfied their lust upon them" (Book 15.23.1.). In part reportedly due to the credence lent this idea by Augustine's examination of it, the notion of incubi became a part of Christian teaching well into the Middle Ages. The female equivalent of the seductive evil spirit was known as a *succubus*, who, in addition to seducing the unwary male sleeper, eventually drained him of his life energy. Since the creatures were often depicted as both seductive and oppressive, they were thought to cause a feeling of weightiness on the chest. Succubi later took on a more alluring seductive character, but in the medieval ages they were portrayed as demonic.

During the medieval Renaissance of the sixteenth century, the German physician Christoph Wirsung (1500-1571) tried to end some of the theological theorizing by scolding "unbelievers" who propagated the idea that nightmares were the result of witchcraft and by developing a more biologic approach to understanding them (21). He believed that nightmares were reflective of current or future physical ailments, and he prescribed a number of remedies that included purges, gargles, stimulants, and dietary changes.

The English physician William Bullein (circa 1520-1576) suggested that those suffering from nightmares should ignore the "supersticious Hypocrites, Infidelles, with charmes, coniurynges [spells] and relickes hangying about the necke, to fraie the Mare" (10). Instead, they should entrust "their sleeping and wakyng to Jesus Christ, that they may live honestlie, goe to bed merily, slepe quietlie, and rise early" (10).

Some observations from the eighteenth and nineteenth centuries regarding dreams deserve note. In "Essay 4: Conception" of his 1785 *Essays on the Intellectual Powers of Man*, the Scottish philosopher Thomas Reid (1710-1796) wrestled with

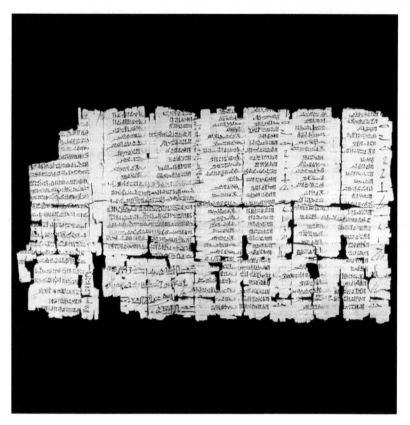

Figure 6 The Dream Book. Understanding the meaning of dreams was a sign of great scholarship in ancient times, and it often garnered significant power for the avid interpreter. In this Egyptian papyri, a list of approximately 108 dreams and their interpretations are inscribed in black (good dreams) or red (bad dreams): "If a man sees himself in a dream looking out of a window, good; it means the hearing of his cry"; or "If a man sees himself in a dream plunging into cold waters, good; it indicates absolution of all ills." Not all dreams were a good omen; for example, a man seeing himself making love to his wife in daylight was a bad omen, suggesting that his god would discover his misdeeds. The high value the Egyptians placed on understanding dreams is also evidenced by the biblical account in Genesis regarding Joseph's interpretations of the Pharoah's troubling dreams: "In the morning his [the Pharaoh's] mind was troubled, so he sent for all the magicians and wise men of Egypt. Pharaoh told them his dreams, but no one could interpret them for him." When Joseph was able to provide an interpretation, he subsequently became a trusted adviser to the Pharaoh (Genesis 41:8, NIV). (Fragments of papyri from Deir el-Medina, Egypt [circa 1279-1213 BC].) (From The Trustees of the British Museum. London. [Used with permission.])

Most early observers of sleep concerned themselves with the purpose of sleep and the meaning of dreams. However, what actually causes sleep, and from whence does it originate? Historically, theories on the mechanics of how we sleep could be categorized in four groups: vascular, chemical, neural, and behavioral (26).

We have already seen how the early philosophers and physicians attributed sleep specifically to divine intervention. However, Alcmaeon (circa sixth and fifth centuries BC), was among the first to speculate on the natural physiology of sleep. He believed that sleep was brought on by blood receding from vessels under the skin to the interior of the body, thus causing immobilization and a lack of sensation (27). Aristotle put forth a chemical and vascular theory, surmising that sleep resided in the heart and was due to the sequelae of "fumes" being absorbed into the blood after the ingestion of food (10). The Roman naturalist Pliny (AD 23-79) wrote in the first century AD that anything without a brain could not sleep, a view later adopted by Galen, who conceptualized sleep as taking place in the brain, which caused it to be temporarily disconnected from the rest of the body (10,19).

Despite the lack of experimental or factual verification, the ever-preeminent Peripatetic views dominated the understanding of sleep until the fifteenth century when the Veronese anatomist Alessandro Benedietti (1452-1512) discovered through careful dissections that almost all nerves originate in the brain. He concluded that sleep takes place in the brain, rather than in the heart as Aristotle had stated. Benedietti faced no less a battle than did Galileo (1564-1642) in overcoming the

supremely entrenched veneration of Aristotle's writings almost a century later. In a work published posthumously in 1520, Bolognese anatomist Alessandro Achillini (1463-1512) (28) elaborated on Benedietti's idea by ascribing sleep to the stoppage of slender arteries in the base of the brain. Vascular theories such as these, sometimes intermixed with chemical or humoral theories, had many notable proponents, and predominated throughout the end of the nineteenth century.

Despite slow progress in the field of sleep research, in 1822 the French physiologist Pierre Flourens (1794-1867), building on the work of Luigi Rolando (1773-1831), showed that bilateral ablation of the cerebral hemispheres of pigeons produced a condition similar to sleep (which we would now call coma) (29). With that finding, the address of sleep was securely assigned to the brain, and neural theories of sleep subsequently predominated.

In 1928, the German neuropsychiatrist Hans Berger recorded the brain's electrical activity and found a distinct difference between waking and sleeping rhythms (30). During an encephalitis epidemic a year later, Constantin von Economo identified specific loci in the brain that seemed responsible for the functions of sleep and alertness while he was studying patients with encephalitis who suffered from excessive sleepiness or pervasive insomnia (ie, encephalitis lethargica) (31) (Figure 10 [32]). In 1935-36, Frédéric Bremer described the characteristic, diagnostic surface electroencephalographic (EEG) findings unique to sleep (33). Then in 1953, Aserinsky and Kleitman (24) published a brief 2-page paper in *Science* on REM and NREM electrical activity that revolutionized both

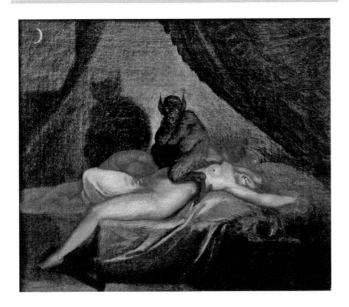

Figure 7 Personification of Nightmare. The sinister dark creature is a weight upon the dreamer, rendering her unable to move. The glowing red eyes and brooding posture of the misshapen creature, along with the frightening shadows, coalesce to convince the viewer that the dreams in this case are not at all pleasant. In rapid eye movement sleep, when our most active and vivid dreams occur, the axial skeletal muscle tone is inhibited, rendering us incapable of movement. Occasionally, when a person partially awakens (from a nightmare or otherwise), there may be a momentary feeling of paralysis, an ofttimes frightening experience called *sleep paralysis.* Frequent bouts of sleep paralysis or the ability to physically act out dreams are often signs of a sleep disorder (see Chapter 9 on "Movement Disorders and Parasomnias"). (Oil on canvas painting titled *Nachtmahr* [*Nightmare*] (1800) by Nicolai Abraham Abildgaard [1743-1809].) (From Danish Museums Online, Denmark.)

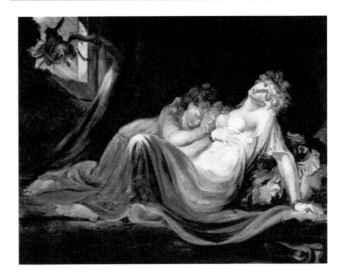

Figure 8 Incubus and Succubus: Special Dreams and Nightmares. In medieval times the incubus was said to be an evil spirit who visited the female sleeper (although occasionally it was depicted as visiting a male sleeper) for the purpose of sexual gratification. Its counterpart, the succubus, was thought be a female spirit that visited and seduced sleeping males. In some tales the succubus consumed the man's energy or life force during intercourse. In later incarnations succubi sometimes were commingled with vampires. (Oil on canvas painting titled *Der Nachtmahr verläßt das Lager zweier schlafender Mädchen [The Nightmare Leaves the Two Sleeping Maidens]* by Johann Heinrich Füssli [1793].) (From Muraltengut, Zurich, Switzerland.)

cognitive and sleep studies and served as conclusive proof that sleep is indeed an active neurological process residing in the brain (Figure 11).

The science of sleep has erupted in recent decades. The biochemical basis of why one becomes sleepy, the genes that determine circadian rhythm, and the discovery of novel neurotransmitter systems that serve an integral function in the delicate balance of wake, NREM, and REM sleep have all been clarified only recently. Current sleep research is no longer confined to philosophy, theology, or psychology but is instead pursued by nearly every discipline of science. There are no fewer than five peer-reviewed international scientific journals dedicated exclusively to sleep, with more venues on the way.

SLEEP DISORDERS

There are persons who have a disposition to sleep on every occasion. They do so at all times, and in all places. They sleep after dinner; they sleep in the theatre, they sleep in church. It is the same to them in what situation they may be placed: sleep is the great end of their existence—their occupation—their sole employment… [these are] our dull, heavy-handed, drowsy mortals,

those sons and daughters of phlegm—with passion as inert as a Dutch fog, and intellects as sluggish as the movements of the hippopotamus or leviathan
(Robert Macnish [7]).

From the beginning, opinions abounded about how to promote good sleep, even while the purpose, origin, and parameters determining the quality of sleep were uncertain. Hippocrates (circa 460-377 BC) recommended sleeping on the left or right side in a cool place, well covered, and with arms, neck, and legs slightly bent (10). Avicenna suggested that sleep should commence on a full stomach (10). The Spanish-born Jewish philosopher Maimonides (AD 1138-1204) recommended eating one's meal three to four hours before going to sleep on one's side, and then switching sides in the middle of the night. The French physician André Du Laurens (1558-1609) ordered his patients to exercise between supper and bedtime; he also dispensed recipes for eight compound internal medicines and 11 outwardly applied medicines as a cure for insomnia (10). Walter Bailey (1529-1592), who served as the physician to Queen Elizabeth I (1533-1603), cautioned against sleeping in a moonlit room because he believed that moonlight bred rheumatic diseases, a recommendation that may have led to the popularity of the canopy bed (10). Bailey also discouraged patients from sleeping for longer than seven hours.

Insomnia is the oldest recorded sleep disorder, as related in the ancient Judaic texts. The biblical figure Job (circa 1000-500 BC) complained, "Nights of misery have been assigned to me. When I lie down I think, 'How long before I get up?' The

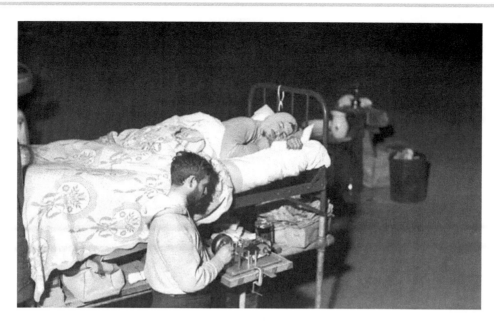

Figure 9 Early Investigations of Sleep. Sleep medicine pioneer Nathaniel Kleitman and his student Eugene Aserinsky were the first to describe rapid eye movement (REM) sleep in humans, starting with observations of their own children. Kleitman also investigated the circadian aspects of sleep on subjects isolated in Kentucky's Mammoth Cave (shown here). (From Mammoth Cave National Park collection [public domain].)

night drags on, and I toss till dawn" (Job 7:3-4; NIV [5]). The ancient Hebrews attributed insomnia to anxiety, stress, or a guilty conscience. Later on in the ancient Greek period, Hippocrates theorized that old age caused what he termed *agrypnia* (sleeplessness) and Pliny recommended sips of "peony in wine" to prevent an attack of what he called *suppressionibus nocturnis*. Insomnia has probably always been the most common sleep disorder, and many remedies have been proposed throughout the ages.

Although less common than insomnia, hypersomnia has also been noted throughout the centuries. Descriptions of sleeping sickness (i.e., African trypanosomiasis) date back centuries (circa AD 1374) to when Sultan Mansa Djata (1360-1374) of Mali died from what was called a *sleeping illness* that "frequently afflicts the inhabitants of that climate" (34). History also documents epidemics of hypersomnia, including an illness that the English physician Thomas Sydenham (1624-1689) called *febris comatosa* that swept London from 1673 to 1675 and the better known encephalitis lethargica outbreak that occurred in Europe and North America from 1916 to 1927, affecting more than one million people and causing a half-million deaths (35).

In retrospect, history also contains vivid examples of more recently defined sleep disorders. For example, the earliest recorded description of what is now referred to as OSA originated around 360 BC. Dionysius (360-305 BC), the massively obese ruler of Heracleaia, fell asleep frequently; to awaken him, servants had to stick sharp needles into his skin and fat (36,37).

> Accordingly, Nymphis of Heraclea, in the second book of his *History of Heraclea*, says—'Dionysius, the son of Clearchus, who was the first tyrant of Heraclia, who was himself afterwards tyrant of his country, grew enormously fat without perceiving

it, owing to his luxury and to his daily gluttony; so that on account of his obesity he was constantly oppressed by a difficulty of breathing and a feeling of suffocation. On which account his physicians ordered thin needles of an exceedingly great length to be made, to be run into his sides and chest whenever he fell into a deeper sleep than usual. . . . and was awakened by them (38).'

The first clinical description of what is now called *complex sleep apnea*, a sleep-related breathing disorder with features of both obstructive and central sleep apnea phenotypes, was probably published in 1877 by Sir William Broadbent. He wrote that in some snoring patients, "every now and then the inspiration fails to overcome the resistance in the pharynx of which stertor or snoring is the audible sign" and he noted in his own patient that "the snoring ceased at regular intervals," whereas other events were not due merely to upper airway obstruction, "but actual cessation of all respiratory movements" (39). Twelve years later, the English physician Richard Caton presented a case to the Clinical Society of London of an obese poulterer who would fall asleep anywhere—even while working:

> He would wake and find himself holding in his hand the duck or chicken which he had been selling to a customer a quarter of an hour before, the customer having at the meantime departed (39).

Caton's full description of the patient shows that the man had severe OSA, which Caton incorrectly called *narcolepsy*, a term coined in 1880 by Jean-Baptiste Edouard Gélineau (1828-1906). What we now know as narcolepsy was actually first

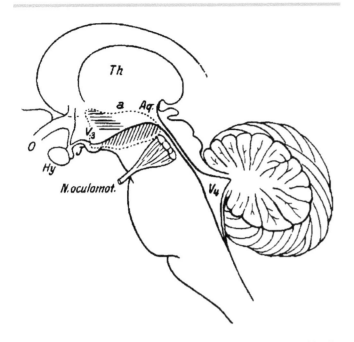

Figure 10 Encephalitis Lethargica. Nearly coincident with the influenza epidemic of 1917, Constantin von Economo described a series of unusual cases characterized by intense hypersomnolence that either worsened after presentation, culminating in coma and death, or gradually improved after 1 to 2 weeks. Less well known is his description of a hyperkinetic form of the disease characterized by severe back and neck pain, weakness, agitation, and insomnia or circadian abnormalities. He proposed the site of the lesion causing prolonged sleepiness as the junction of the brainstem and forebrain (diagonal hatching) and the site of the lesion causing insomnia as the anterior hypothalamus (horizontal hatching). Von Economo's investigation was a foundational step toward understanding the neurobiology of sleep. The "a" indicates dotted line boundary containing the field that Von Economo found important in the regulation of sleep; Aq, aqueduct; Hy, hypophysis; J, infundibulum; *N. oculamot.*, nervus oculomotorius; O, optic chiasm; Th, optical thalamus; V_3, third ventricle; and V_4, fourth ventricle. (Line drawing from von Economo [32]. [Used with permission.])

identified in 1877 by Karl Friedrich Otto Westphal (1833-1890) (40).

The identification and naming of the condition that came to be called the *Pickwickian syndrome* is a popular topic in the history of sleep medicine and will be discussed further in Chapter 6. The term derives from the vivid description by Charles Dickens of a fat boy named Joe in his serialized novel *The Posthumous Papers of the Pickwick Club* published in 1836-1837 (Figure 12). Somnolence, hypoventilation, and obesity were first linked in the medical literature as a disorder called Pickwickian syndrome in a 1956 report by C. Sidney Burwell. However, William Shakespeare (1564-1616) probably deserves credit for an earlier description, albeit literary, of the clinical features of OSA in his portrayal of the rotund Falstaff (Figure 13) in his plays, including *King Henry IV*:

Falstaff:	Now, Hal, what time of day is it, lad?
Prince Henry:	Thou art so fat-witted, with drinking of old sack, and unbuttoning thee after supper and sleeping upon benches after noon.... (act 1, scene 2)
Peto:	Falstaff! Fast asleep behind the arras, and snorting like a horse.
Prince Henry:	Hark, how hard he fetches breath.... (act 2, scene 4)

The OSA syndrome as we define it today was first medically reported at a conference in 1965 by Henri Gastaut and colleagues, who explained it as an interruption of activity in the respiratory center (41). Audience members Richard Jung and Wolfgang Kuhl were intrigued enough to conduct further research and attributed OSA to an intermittent blockage of the upper airways.

The pattern of central sleep apnea that is best recognized is named Cheyne-Stokes respiration after the two men who first observed and described it. The initial observation by John Cheyne (1777-1836) of the rhythmic cessation of breathing was eventually published more than 30 years later in 1854 by William Stokes:

> The decline in the length and force of the respirations is as regular and remarkable as their progressive increase. The inspirations become each one less deep than the preceding, until they are all but

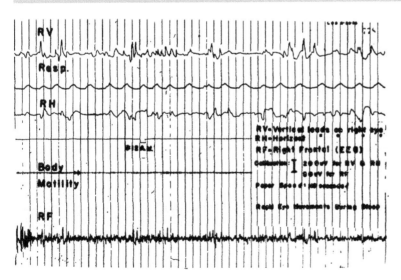

Figure 11 Electroencephalographic Activity During Sleep. In the first report of rapid eye movement (REM) in a sleeping person in 1953, Aserinsky and Kleitman (24) used electro-oculogram tracings (first and third lines from top) to document REM in the right eye of a sleeper (calibration 200 microvolts for RV and RH and 50 microvolts for RF; paper speed, 10 seconds). Resp, respiration; RF, right frontal electroencephalogram; RH, horizontal leads on right eye; RV, vertical leads on right eye. (From Aserinsky and Kleitman [24]. [Used with permission.])

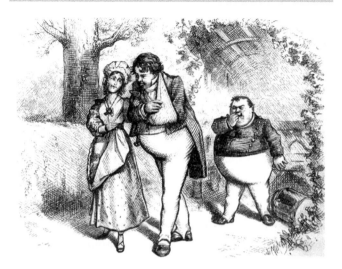

Figure 12 Joe—The Fat Boy. An illustration by Thomas Nast of the obese minor character Joe appeared in the book-length version of *The Posthumous Papers of the Pickwick Club* by Charles Dickens (first published in serial form between March 1836 and October 1837). The description of Joe as a perennially sleepy servant who falls asleep anytime he is not eating has led sleep experts to diagnose Joe's condition as resulting from impaired sleep due to obstructive sleep apnea. (From Dickens C. The Posthumous Papers of the Pickwick Club. New York: Harper and Brothers, 1873.)

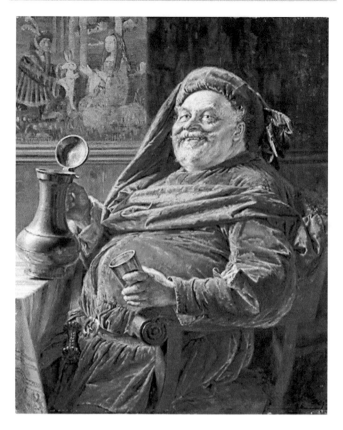

Figure 13 Obesity and Obstructive Sleep Apnea. The English playwright William Shakespeare often portrayed an obese character, a favorite in literature for his wit and roguery. One such character was Falstaff, who was known for his somnolent tendencies and his loud snoring, both symptoms of obstructive sleep apnea. These qualities, no doubt familiar to all observers of the human condition, are portrayed in musical form in Edward Elgar's *Falstaff*, Symphonic study in C minor, Op. 68. There, in the second movement, Eastcheap, the bassoon, portrays the corpulent snoring form of Falstaff. In another musical rendition of *Falstaff* (1799), Antonio Salieri also highlighted the snoring and sleeping form. (Oil painting on canvas titled *Falstaff mit großer Weinkanne und Becher* [*Falstaff With Large Wine Can and Cup*] [1896] by Eduard von Grützner.)

imperceptible; and then the state of apparent apnoea occurs. This is at last broken by the faintest possible inspiration: the next effort is a little stronger, until, so to speak, the paroxysm of breathing is at its height, again to subside by a descending scale! (42)

Although Hippocrates is thought to have also alluded to this same breathing pattern in sleepers, the most vivid description was made in 1781 by John Hunter (1728-1793), preceding Cheyne's report by 37 years:

His breathing was very particular: he would cease breathing for twenty or thirty seconds, and then begin to breathe softly, which increased until he breathed extremely strong, or rather with violent strength, which gradually died away till we could not observe that he breathed at all (43).

Thus a case for naming it "Hunter respirations" could be advanced with some merit.

The developments in understanding sleep apnea, coupled with the discovery of REM sleep, produced burgeoning interest in sleep medicine as a clinical field (Table 2). The germination of the European Sleep Research Society probably occurred during a well-attended electroencephalography conference organized by Henri Gastaut and Elio Lugaresi that was held in Bologna, Italy, in 1967 (proceedings published as *The Abnormalities of Sleep in Man*). The formation of the European Sleep Research Society was completed during a meeting organized by U. J. Jovanović and held in Würzburg in 1971. Meanwhile, in 1970 Stanford University launched the world's first sleep disorders clinic, which produced rapid developments in diagnostic and therapeutic techniques, as well as in research (41). In 1972, the same year that treatments for OSA were described, a sleep conference on "Hypersomnia With Periodic Breathing" was held in Rimini, Italy, sparking international interest in sleep research (50). In the United States, the Association of Sleep Disorders Centers (now the American Academy of Sleep Medicine) was started in 1975, and in 1989 the first sleep medicine textbook (47) was published. In the ongoing maturation process, the specialty of sleep medicine, no longer an awkward progeny of several feeder sciences and specialties, was admitted to the American Board of Medical Specialties, and the first American Board of Medical Specialties Examination in Sleep Medicine was offered in fall 2007.

Table 2 Landmarks in sleep medicine

Year	Landmark
1781	Periodic breathing is described by John Hunter
1854	William Stokes (44) publishes a description of the respiration pattern common in central sleep apnea (Cheyne-Stokes respiration), as observed by John Cheyne 30 years earlier
1880	Narcolepsy is first named by Jean-Baptiste Edouard Gélineau
1889	First medical description of obstructive sleep apnea syndrome is given by Richard Caton, speaking to the Clinical Society of London
1939	Nathaniel Kleitman publishes *Sleep and Wakefulness* (45)
1964	Stanford Narcolepsy Center is founded
1964	Henri Gastaut presents a polysomnographically complete picture of obstructive sleep apnea (published in 1965)
1965	Sleeping pills are evaluated using polysomnography
1967	International conference on sleep disorders is held, the proceedings of which are published as *The Abnormalities of Sleep in Man* (46)
1968	Manual for scoring sleep is developed
1970	Effectiveness of tracheostomy for treatment of obstructive sleep apnea is reported by Lugaresi and colleagues
1972	Respiratory and cardiac monitors enter routine use with polysomnography, thus increasing awareness of obstructive sleep apnea
1972	First academic course is offered on "The Diagnosis and Treatment of Sleep Disorders" (a 1-day course at Stanford University)
1975	Association of Sleep Disorders is established, with five centers as charter members
1975	Polysomnography is deemed a medical test worthy of financial reimbursement by third-party payers in the U.S.
1976	Multiple Sleep Latency Test is developed by Mary Carskadon to quantify degrees of sleepiness
1978	Specialty journal *Sleep* is launched
1981	Continuous positive airway pressure is described by Colin Sullivan and colleagues as a nonsurgical treatment for obstructive sleep apnea
1987	American Sleep Disorders Association is founded
1989	First textbook of sleep medicine, the *Principles and Practice of Sleep Medicine* by Meir Kryger and colleagues (47), is published
1991	American Board of Sleep Medicine is founded; first edition of *The International Classification of Sleep Disorders* (ICSD) (48) is published
1999	American Academy of Sleep Medicine replaces the American Board of Sleep Medicine
2003	Behavioral Sleep Medicine Certification is initiated
2005	Second edition of the *International Classification of Sleep Disorders* (ICSD-2) (49) is published; specialty journal *Clinical Sleep Medicine* is launched
2007	Examination for sleep medicine board certification is offered under the parent organization, the American Board of Medical Subspecialties

REFERENCES

1. Gordon NP, Clearly PD, Parker CE, Czeisler CA. The prevalence and health impact of shiftwork. Am J Public Health 1986; 76: 1225–8.
2. The Iliad of Homer. Trans. Alexander Pope. London: Grant Richards, 1902.
3. Genesis 2:21 (New King James Version).
4. Buhler G. Indian History Sourcebook: The Laws of Manu, c. 1500 BCE [Internet] [cited 2009 Oct 27]. Available from: http://www.fordham.edu/halsall/india/manu-full.html.
5. Judges 16:19 (New International Version).
6. Butcher SH, Lang M. The Odyssey of Homer. New York: The Macmillan Co., 1900.
7. Macnish R. The Philosophy of Sleep. New York: D. Appleton, 1834.
8. Lavie P. The Enchanted World of Sleep. Trans. Anthony Berris. New Haven (CT): Yale University Press, 1996.
9. Gallop D, editor. Aristotle on Sleep and Dreams: A Text and Translation With Introduction, Notes, and Glossary. Warminster (England): Aris & Phillips, 1996.
10. Dannenfeldt KH. Sleep: theory and practice in the late Renaissance. J Hist Med Allied Sci 1986; 41: 415–41.
11. Lavie P, Hobson JA. Origin of dreams: anticipation of modern theories in the philosophy and physiology of the eighteenth and nineteenth centuries. Psychol Bull 1986; 100: 229–40.
12. Siegel JM. Clues to the functions of mammalian sleep. Nature 2005; 437: 1264–71.
13. Gottesmann C. The golden age of rapid eye movement sleep discoveries. 1. Lucretius: 1964. Prog Neurobiol 2001; 65: 211–87.
14. Meier C. Caesar: A Biography. MJF Books, 2003.
15. Holowchak MA. Interpreting dreams for corrective regimen: diagnostic dreams in Greco-Roman medicine. J Hist Med Allied Sci 2001; 56: 382–99.
16. Hippocrates. Trans. William Henry Samuel Jones. Cambridge (MA): Harvard University Press, 1984.
17. Adler RE. Medical Firsts: From Hippocrates to the Human Genome. Hoboken (NJ): John Wiley & Sons, 2004.
18. Artemidorus. Interpretation of Dreams: Oneirocritica. 2nd ed. Original Books, 1990.
19. Oberhelman SM. Galen: on diagnosis from dreams. J Hist Med Allied Sci 1983; 38: 36–47.
20. St. Augustine. Concerning the City of God Against the Pagans. Trans. Henry Bettenson. New York (NY): Penguin Books, 2003.
21. Wirsung C. Praxis Medicine Universalis. Londoni: Impensis Georg. Bishop, 1598.
22. Reid T. Essays on the Intellectual Powers of Man [Internet] [cited 2009 Oct 27], p. 799. Available from: http://www.earlymodern texts.com/f_reid.html.
23. Freud S. The Interpretation of Dreams. In: Strachey J, editor and translator. The Standard Edition of the Complete Psychological Works of Sigmund Freud. Vol. 4-5 (1900). London: Hogarth Press, 1953.
24. Aserinsky E, Kleitman N. Regularly occurring periods of eye motility, and concomitant phenomena, during sleep. Science 1953; 118: 273–74.
25. The Confessions of St. Augustine. Trans. EB Pusey. New York: EP Dutton and Co., 1907.
26. Thorpy MJ. The Encyclopedia of Sleep and Sleep Disorders. New York: Facts on File, 1991.
27. Lavie P. Restless Nights: Understanding Snoring and Sleep Apnea. New Haven: Yale University Press, 2003.
28. Achillini A. Annotationes Anatomiae. Bonon: Per Hieronymum de Benedictis, 1520.
29. Finger S. Origins of Neuroscience: A History of Explorations Into Brain Function. New York: Oxford University Press, 1994.

30. Berger H. Über das electroenkphalogramm des menschen. J Psychol Neurol 1930; 40: 160–79.

31. Reid AH, McCall S, Henry JM, Taubenberger JK. Experimenting on the past: the enigma of von Economo's encephalitis lethargica. J Neuropathol Exp Neurol 2001; 60: 663–70.

32. v. Economo C. Sleep as a problem of localization. J Nerv Ment Dis 1930; 71: 249–59.

33. Kerkhofs M, Lavie P. Frederic Bremer 1892-1982: a pioneer in sleep research. Sleep Med Rev 2000; 4: 505–14.

34. Cox FE. History of sleeping sickness (African trypanosomiasis). Infect Dis Clin North Am 2004; 18: 231–45.

35. Triarhou LC. The percipient observations of Constantin von Economo on encephalitis lethargica and sleep disruption and their lasting impact on contemporary sleep research. Brain Res Bull 2006; 69: 244–58. Epub 2006 Mar 3.

36. Bray GA. What's in a name? Mr. Dickens' "Pickwickian" fat boy syndrome. Obes Res 1994; 2: 380–83.

37. Kryger MH. Sleep apnea: from the needles of Dionysius to continuous positive airway pressure. Arch Intern Med 1983; 143: 2301–3.

38. Athenaesus, of Naucratis. The Deipnosophists. Trans. Charles Duke Yonge. London: HG Bohn, 1853-54.

39. Lavie P. Nothing new under the moon: historical accounts of sleep apnea syndrome. Arch Intern Med 1984; 144: 2025–8.

40. Schenck CH, Bassetti CL, Arnulf I, Mignot E. English translations of the first clinical reports on narcolepsy and cataplexy by Westphal and Gelineau in the last 19th century, with commentary. J Clin Sleep Med 2007; 3: 301–11.

41. Dement WC. History of sleep medicine. Neurol Clin 2005; 23: 945–65.

42. Lavie P. Restless Nights: Understanding Snoring and Sleep Apnea. Trans. Anthony Berris. New Haven: Yale University Press, 2003.

43. Ward M. Periodic respiration: a short historical note. Ann R Coll Surg Engl 1973; 52: 330–4.

44. Stokes W. The Diseases of the Heart and the Aorta. Philadelphia: Lindsay and Blakiston: 1854.

45. Kleitman N. Sleep and Wakefulness as Alternating Phases in the Cycle of Existence. Chicago: University of Chicago Press, 1939.

46. Gastaut H, editor. The Abnormalities of Sleep in Man. Proceedings of the 15th European Meeting on Electroencephalography, 1967; Bologna, Italy; 1968.

47. Kryger MH, Roth T, Dement WC, editors. Principles and Practice of Sleep Medicine. Philadelphia: Saunders, 1989.

48. Thorpy MJ, American Sleep Disorders Association, Diagnostic Classification Steering Committee. The International Classification of Sleep Disorders: Diagnostic and Coding Manual. Rochester (MN): American Sleep Disorders Association, 1991.

49. American Academy of Sleep Medicine. The International Classification of Sleep Disorders: Diagnostic and Coding Manual. 2nd ed. Westchester (IL): American Academy of Sleep Medicine, 2005.

50. Sadoul P, Lugaresi E, editors. Hypersomnia with periodic breathing: symposium. Bull Physiopathologie Respiratoire 1972; 8: 967–1292.

2

Cross-Cultural Aspects of Sleep

Lois E. Krahn, MD

Culture is considered to be the patterns of behavior, norms, and shared experiences among the members of a group of people. This chapter explores how cultural practices influence sleep by identifying and exploring 1) the cultural factors that predispose to healthy and unhealthy sleep, 2) the cultural explanations for sleep complaints, and 3) the traditional treatments for sleep disorders that are used in different cultural settings. Given all the cultures and subcultures within the global community, this chapter is necessarily limited to select examples that illustrate the main points of this fascinating but less well-studied topic.

CULTURAL PRACTICES THAT INFLUENCE SLEEP

Cultural issues are especially relevant to understanding insomnia and disorders of circadian rhythm, conditions in which the patient's interaction with the sleep environment with respect to timing and comfort is especially influential. This chapter is divided into sections that describe important aspects of sleep environment and scheduling that influence sleep duration, quality, and synchronization with the community.

The quality and duration of sleep are greatly influenced by cultural practices that may determine the sleep environment (e.g., bedding or location of bed), sleep schedule, duration of sleep, nap schedule, and customs that increase the risk for specific sleep disorders.

Sleep Environment

Over the millennia, beds have varied in shape and size (1). From the relics found in the tomb of Tutankhamen (circa 1370-1352 BC), it is apparent that the bed of a wealthy Egyptian royal family member was an elaborate and comfortable place to sleep (Figure 1). In the ancient Greek and Roman cultures, people of sufficient wealth slept on wooden couches that were also used for eating (Figure 2). In Rome, depending on the person's means, these couches might be topped with a mattress made of straw, reeds, herbs, wool, feathers, or swan down. Canopies, curtains, and mosquito nets were added to provide warmth, privacy, and protection from insects. For many centuries, bedding remained basically unchanged. By the Tudor era in England (1485-1603), beds had evolved into elegant pieces of furniture decorated with ornate carvings and draped with heavy curtains. The bedchamber became the accepted site for publicly celebrated ceremonies such as receiving guests, as well as births, marriages, and deaths (Figure 3). Later a style of bedding was adopted in northern Europe that utilized cupboards to optimize privacy and warmth (Figure 4).

For the working class, beds evolved from bundles of straw on the ground shared by whole families. Native American Indians used a woven mat to demarcate the sleeping area of their dwelling (Figure 5). Animal hides were used to provide warmth. Harsh climatic conditions, such as in the polar regions, required the Eskimo (Inuit) people to adopt specialized bedding made of animal fur and elevated from the ground to conserve body heat (Figure 6). In warmer regions, efforts to provide a sufficiently cool sleeping environment were necessary by optimizing ventilation and airflow (Figure 7). Bedding sometimes evolved that did not incorporate comfortable materials, for example, the rigid pillow used by some African tribes (Figure 8).

Over the centuries, comfortable mattresses were more fully upgraded by using cloth bags stuffed with rags and pieces of wool and were eventually placed on simple wooden platforms rather than the floor. Beds were prized possessions, representing a large proportion of a family's assets, and were passed down throughout the generations as bequests. Bedbugs were a hazard until bedding materials could be thoroughly cleaned by boiling them. By the time of the industrial revolution in the late 18th century, beds were more available and the working class had beds that consisted of basic mattresses on frames. After the long-time use of natural filler materials such as straw, feathers, rags, cotton, or wool, technological advances led to the placement of springs inside mattresses in the mid 1850s. Since then innumerable types of spring mattresses have been developed that combine natural or synthetic foams to add layers of comfort. Further innovation over the next 150 years led to mattresses filled with latex foam or water and to mattresses with electronically programmable degrees of firmness.

In more geographically isolated societies such as that of Japan, bedding developed along distinct cultural lines, with *tatami* mats being adopted to provide a softer surface than wood (Figure 9). Tatami mats consisted of compressed rice straw (*doko*) covered by layers of paper, woven rush grass (*omote*), and cloth (*heri*). In the 17th century, wealthy Japanese placed a mattress stuffed with cotton (*futon*) on top of the tatami. The Japanese used a characteristic pillow, presumably to enhance comfort (Figure 10). In Japanese port communities, futons might be stuffed with seaweed rather than cotton. The loft in the futon was preserved by airing it regularly.

In geographic areas around the world where sleeping on the ground posed risks of exposure to vermin (e.g., Venezuela), a sling-type bed was made of netting or cloth and suspended from each end (i.e., the hammock) (Figure 11). Some cultural groups functioned for centuries with minimal or no bedding.

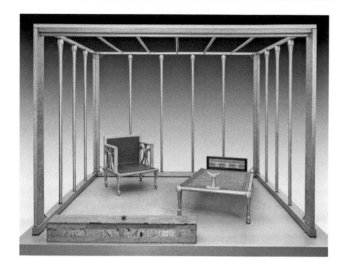

Figure 1 The Egyptians designed impressive beds raised from the floor that were meant to provide comfort and convey the social status or class of the bed's occupant. Egyptian bed (reproduction) from tomb of Queen Hetepheres I (circa 2582-2575 BC) made of wood, gold, copper, silver, leather, faience (glazed earthenware), and ebony. (Photograph © 2010, Museum of Fine Arts, Boston [Used with permission.])

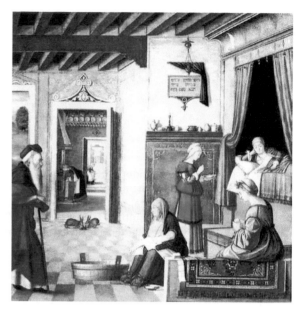

Figure 3 Beds in the Tudor era (1550-1603) were intended to provide privacy but also to allow the bedchamber to be used for special occasions, such as entertaining guests. Elaborate Tudor bed (at right) draped with curtains depicted in the oil painting *The Birth of the Virgin* (1504) by Vittore Carpaccio. (From Bergamo/Accademia Carrara 81LC00235. [Used with permission.])

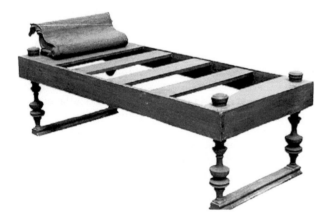

Figure 2 The Romans placed a high value on regal yet comfortable bedding. Roman couch or bed (reproduction) with bronze fittings and wooden body and slats that would have been covered with a cushion. (From Roma, Museo della Civilta Romana. [Used with permission.])

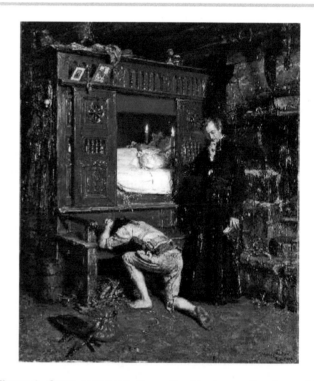

The Efe pygmies in Zaire slept on a thin layer of leaves on the ground whereas the !Kung of Botswana slept directly on the ground (2).

Sleep-Wake Schedule

Sleeping patterns and schedules vary widely across cultures. Steger and Brunt (3) developed a framework to assist with the classification of cultural differences in sleeping patterns from

Figure 4 Some societies further refined beds over time to provide increased warmth and privacy. French cupboard bed depicted in the oil painting *Le Retour* (The Return) (circa 1883) by Henry Mosler. (From Musée départemental Breton, Quimper, France.)

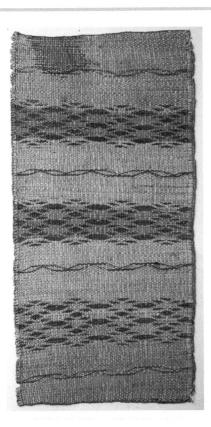

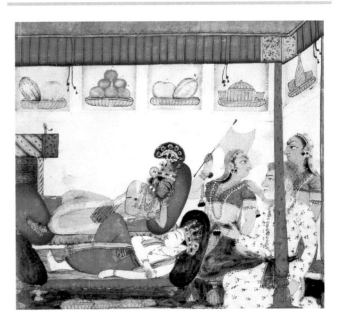

Figure 7 In warm and humid climates, a comfortable sleeping environment required the means to ensure an adequate air flow. Sleeping habits in India depicted in the watercolor *Krishna and Balarama, Watched Over by Nanda and Yashoda, Who Fans Them to Sleep* (circa 1725). (Courtesy of Francesca Galloway, London. [Used with permission.])

Figure 5 Nomadic cultural groups required bedding that was portable and could be constructed from local materials. Woven sleeping mat (circa 1880) of Ojibwa People of North America made from rosewood and reeds and dyed with vegetable dye. (From Museum of International Folk Art, Santa Fe, NM. Gift of Lloyd Cotson and the Neutrogena Corporation. Photo by Pat Pollard. [Used with permission.])

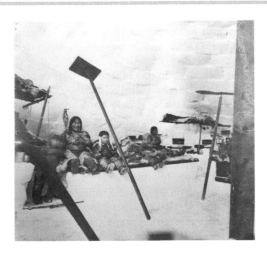

Figure 6 Harsh climatic conditions in the globe's polar regions require modification to preserve body heat. Inuit sleeping arrangements inside an ice igloo include an elevated sleeping bench covered by fur. (Interior of Harry's Snowhouse in the Northwest Territories/Nunavut. Harry was Chief of the Aivilingmiut at Cape Fullerton. Courtesy © Canadian Museum of Civilization, Quebec, Canada [photograph by A. P. Low, 1903, image 2904]. [Used with permission.])

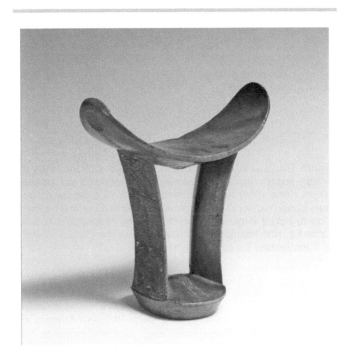

Figure 8 For some cultural groups, bedding materials are viewed as a means to promote both sleep and spiritual needs. African pillows (circa 1950) were headrests made from wood and sometimes decorated with beads. (From The Metropolitan Museum of Art/Art Resource, New York. [Used with permission.])

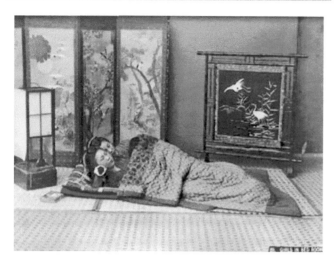

Figure 9 Japanese tatami mat with futon is depicted in photograph, *Girls in Bed Room* (circa 1880). (From Philipp March Old Japan Photography, Bern, Switzerland.)

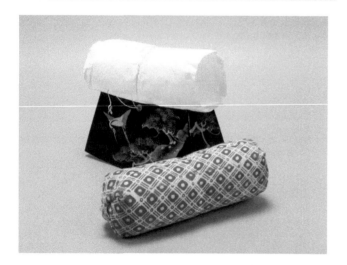

Figure 10 Japanese bedding developed along distinct lines that include specific mattress materials and other features. Japanese pillows (circa 1950) were headrests made from a lacquered wood base topped with a cylindrical pillow wrapped in paper and tied to the base to hold it in place. (From Museum of International Folk Art, Sante Fe, NM. International Folk Art Foundation Collection. Photo by Paul Smutko. [Used with permission.])

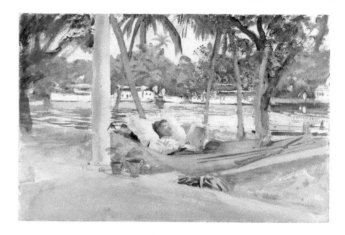

Figure 11 *Figure in Hammock, Florida* (1917 by John Singer Sargent). (From The Metropolitan Museum of Art/Art Resource, New York. [Used with permission.])

no daytime napping to polyphasic sleep. In North America and northern Europe, a monophasic sleep pattern is common. This entails one major nighttime sleep period that lasts eight hours. In contrast, a biphasic sleep pattern is common in Spain and former Spanish colonies that includes a major nocturnal sleep period and a shorter scheduled afternoon nap called a *siesta* that lasts about two hours. The term is derived from the Latin word *sexta* for the sixth hour (i.e., noon), and it means an afternoon rest. The siesta is sometimes thought to have evolved

because of a desire to escape the heat of the day. However, the siesta's association with heat and climate is not absolute because siestas were practiced in northern Europe until the industrial revolution; today they are common in some Chinese communities but largely absent in Portugal. The sleep obtained during the siesta permits activities to continue later into the evening than those which are observed in monophasic cultures. In both the monophasic and biphasic patterns, the need to sleep takes priority. Traditionally, the siesta sleeper dons pajamas and sleeps in bed in a manner similar to that for nighttime sleep. In biphasic cultures, community activities are largely scheduled to avoid night and siesta sleep times (Figure 12).

The third variant, the polyphasic pattern, occurs around the globe, and it entails people napping during the day at will. The societies of Japan and India both have polyphasic sleep patterns. The nap schedule is flexible, depending on the degree of sleepiness and the opportunity to sleep. The primary nocturnal sleep period still satisfies most of the sleep debt, but the community is accepting of people sleeping during the day in many public settings. In Japan the widespread practice of sleeping in public places is called *inemuri*. It is viewed as evidence that persons have made hard work a priority and that they have an overarching commitment to their career or schoolwork. To satisfy their basic sleep needs, people take these brief naps whenever and wherever possible. These spontaneous episodes of sleep allow people to stay up later at night to study or work. One study found that 65% of Japanese men and 71% of Japanese women sleep while riding on trains, a situation that is facilitated by long commuting times (4). Although opportunistic napping is acceptable, the sleep environment is often less private and less conducive to sleep. Japan has been hailed as the noisiest nation on earth, with loudspeakers, buzzers, and sirens creating a nearly continuous stream of noise. No laws exist that place limits on sound amplification, even in residential neighborhoods.

In this era of globalization, these simplified patterns of sleep-wake activity are in transition. North American and European societies are becoming more accepting of the benefits of a brief daytime "power nap" to enhance subsequent alertness. Spain and Japan are increasingly conforming to the

Sleep Schedules of Different Cultural Groups

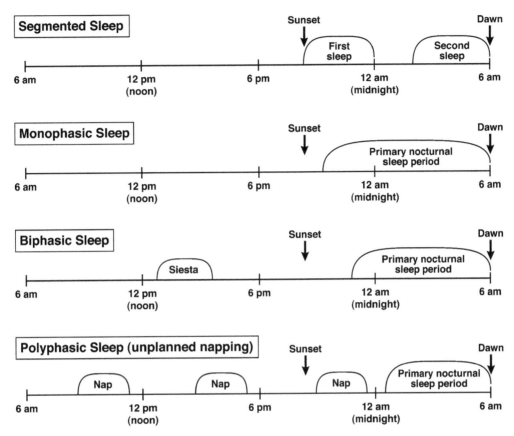

Figure 12 Sleep schedules of different cultural groups around the world based on Steger and Brunt's classification of sleep schedules (3).

conventional workday that precludes an opportunity for a planned siesta or an unplanned nap.

The timing of the major sleep period is culturally determined as well. In the desert of the Arabian peninsula, the workday starts earlier, particularly for outdoor laborers in the summer. Bedtime is advanced accordingly. Year round in traditional Brazilian society, dinner is eaten at 11:00 PM, with bedtime following several hours later. Nonetheless, Brazilians have adequate time for nighttime sleep because daytime activities start later in the morning than they do in northern European and North American countries. The siesta is not practiced in traditional Brazilian society.

Seasonal variations in sleep patterns are especially common at higher latitudes. In the Northern Hemisphere, the sleep period of the Inuit people is relatively restricted during extended daylight hours in the summer but lengthened to as long as 14 hours during the darkness of winter.

Cultural preferences may at times explain a patient's failure to adhere to conventional medical advice or to implement techniques suggested by patient education materials about healthy sleep practices. For example, a patient from Brazil, where dinner is customarily served late in the evening, may not readily accept a recommendation for an earlier bedtime to ensure adequate sleep. The sleep clinician may

therefore be more effective by discussing the need for adequate sleep, which the patient can perhaps obtain by sleeping in later in the morning, rather than by asking the patient to give up an important social activity for sleep. The lack of adherence to sleep hygiene recommendations made by conventional sleep specialists because of the patient's cultural preferences has not been well studied.

Within the sphere of the cross-cultural aspects of sleep, one complication occurs when a person's sleep behaviors do not reflect the practices of others within the surrounding community. In these situations, the divergence of the person's practices from those of the community at large increases the risk for problematic sleep patterns. For example, a Muslim who is observing the month of Ramadan while living in the Middle East will reflect the practices of the majority culture; thus, for a month, he or she can fast and nap during the day while feasting and celebrating every night. Such communities typically reduce the duration of the workday during this period to permit culturally acceptable napping. However, an observant Muslim who is living in the culturally diverse setting of Europe or North America will have no daytime accommodation and thus may struggle more with problematic sleep issues during Ramadan. Nonetheless, even in the case of a Muslim living in the Middle East, the practice of Ramadan that encourages daytime napping at a time when meals would typically be consumed may conflict with human physiologic needs and result in poor sleep quality.

Immigrants, particularly refugee groups, provide a specific example of the challenges of acculturation. A recent study examining new Sudanese immigrants to Canada found that those whose expectations were unfulfilled or who were experiencing economic hardship were 3 to 4 times as likely to have insomnia or to feel stress and sadness as those whose transition was less difficult (5).

CULTURAL EXPLANATIONS OF SLEEP COMPLAINTS

When patients experience a problem with sleep, whether it be insomnia, excessive sleep, or unusual behaviors at night, they usually seek to determine the cause and then to understand its meaning. When there is no clear medical reason for an inability to sleep, such as because of pain, some persons within specific cultural communities may seek other causes, even looking to their beliefs for guidance. Clinicians can best support such patients by becoming knowledgeable about how a community viewed sleep in the past compared with the present; such information may be accessed through various sources that range from art and literature to the Internet.

The development of ayurvedic medicine more than five thousand years ago was based on the theory that, vital energy—referred to as *prana*—is the basis of all life and healing. As prana circulates throughout the human body, it is governed by the five elements: earth, air, fire, water, and ether. Health, a state of balance and harmony among the five elements, is referred to as a person's *prakriti* (i.e., constitution). Illness occurs when there is imbalance or lack of harmony among them. This philosophy recognizes the importance of chronobiology. The five elements combine with one another into pairs called *doshas*. The three doshas are *vata* (ether and air), *pitta* (fire and water), and *kapha* (earth and water). Illness is perceived in terms of how the doshas are out of balance in comparison with the prakriti. The three doshas have specific roles in a person's daily rhythm. Ayurvedic medicine holds that each 24-hour cycle is divided into 4-hour segments that are governed by the doshas (Table 1). In turn, the daily cycles of the three doshas are synchronized with the configuration of the sun, moon, earth, and planets in the solar system. These time periods are believed to correspond with nature and to dictate optimal times for certain functions such as exercise, work, rest, digestion, fasting, or healing. Each dosha can become imbalanced by an unhealthy lifestyle, poor diet, excessive activity, minimal activity, and external factors such as germs or weather. Of the three doshas, the vata is the most relevant to sleep. For example, imbalance can be caused by staying up late at night, which is thought to trigger skin, neurological, and mental disorders. A

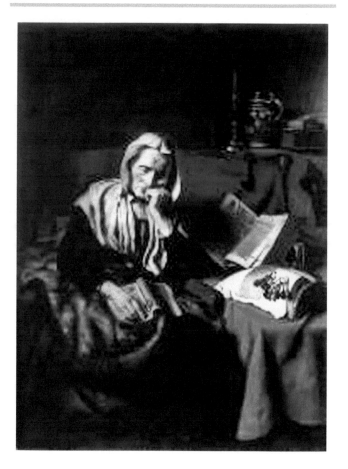

Figure 13 The societal view of sleep, and daytime napping in particular, has changed over the years to a more favorable one. *Old Woman Dozing* (circa 1655) by the Dutch baroque portraitist Nicolaes Maes. (From Musées Royaux des Beaux-Arts de Belgique, Brussels, Belgium. [Used with permission.])

healthy person wakes up before 6:00 AM, ideally between 4:30 and 5:00 AM, before the end of the vata dosha, which corresponds with sunrise. Bedtime is at 10:00 PM, which corresponds with the start of the pitta dosha. Adherence to this sleep-wake schedule allows for 6 to 7 hours of sleep time.

Another example of how a specific cultural group views sleep and how these beliefs change over the centuries comes from northern Europe. Several 17th century Dutch paintings depict a sleeping person, including *Old Woman Dozing* by Nicolaes Maes (Figure 13). The woman sleeps with her lace bobbins nearby (a symbol of productivity) and two open books, one of which is a Bible. It is believed that such paintings were intended to convey a warning against idleness or a message that sleep renders a person vulnerable to danger or, if alcohol is depicted, a caution against the risks of excessive alcohol use. Sleeping during the day was considered sinful for people of all ages. For an older person, sleep was viewed as an even greater waste of time because such persons have a shortened life expectancy. In this painting, an hourglass is depicted, which symbolizes that time (i.e., life) is running out, and the Bible is open to the book of Amos, the "prophet of doom" who warns about moral depravity. Assuming that Maes' message reflected the values of 17th century Dutch society, the need to nap during the day must not have been acceptable (6).

Table 1 Three doshas of ayurvedic medicine that complete two cycles during a 24-hour day

Dosha	Elements	Timing
Vata	Space and air	2:00 PM to 6:00 PM 2:00 AM to 6:00 AM
Kapha	Water and earth	6:00 AM to 10:00 AM 6:00 PM to 10:00 PM
Pitta	Fire and water	10:00 AM to 2:00 PM 10:00 PM to 2:00 AM

Insomnia is the predominant feature of a condition called *Hwa-Byung* that is found in the Korean culture. This term translates as "anger sickness." Traditional healers observe an excessive fire (i.e., anger) relative to the other four universal elements within ancient Asian medicine (i.e., earth, water, wood, and metal). Patients will typically have epigastric pain initially that they fear will cause their death. These symptoms are closely associated with insomnia, fatigue, and other pain complaints. The condition generally develops in women with traditional beliefs who become assertive and subsequently face stressful circumstances such as a strained marriage. With its symptoms of depressed mood and anxiety, this condition is similar to the somatoform disorder diagnosed in Western medicine. Polysomnography reveals alpha intrusion into slow-wave sleep. Traditional treatment involves various combinations of Chinese herbs. Conventional treatment provided by health care providers includes various expressive psychotherapies that help the patient to express anger, improve quality of life, and reduce symptom intensity (7).

Insomnia is one of the symptoms of an illness called *susto*, a condition found among persons in the Mexican-American culture. When a person dreams while asleep, the spirit supposedly leaves the body to wander far and wide. If the spirit is not near enough to the body to reenter when needed, its absence can lead to insomnia, irritability, anorexia, and anxiety. A related but more serious condition is *espanto*, which is the loss of spirit caused by being awakened by something frightening, such as a natural disaster, falling out of bed, or a nightmare (8).

From a cross-cultural standpoint, sleep paralysis has been studied more than other sleep conditions. Sleep paralysis can be a frightening experience because the inability to move is often coupled with dreaming that persists as the patient progressively awakens. To explain this phenomenon, patients may turn to plausible events in their life experience. The Inuit people call sleep paralysis *uqumangirniq* or *aqtuqsinniq*, depending on their geographic region within the polar region. Older Inuit people explain these phenomena with the belief that the person's soul was vulnerable during sleep and dreaming and thus was subjected to an attack by evil spirits. This older group interprets the lack of control over sleep paralysis by turning to supernatural beliefs that themselves serve as evidence of such spirits. However, Inuit society is modernizing and younger persons have identified several more quantifiable factors that may contribute to sleep paralysis, including personal, medical, mystical, traditional, and Christian factors (9).

In Nigeria, a similar condition of *ogun oru* (also known as nocturnal warfare) is attributed to demonic possession of a person while dreaming. Traditional healers assess the patient by hearing a description, observing the patient, and conducting divination. The features of ogun oru include being attacked at night while asleep or being poisoned by an enemy while dreaming about eating. The patient then awakens and is unable to fall asleep again. The patient may become agitated, usually at night but sometimes during the day. The dreams are not typically recalled by the patient because of spiritual concealment but are only identified by the traditional healer in the course of the assessment. A recent paper described three cases of ogun oru in three women ranging in age from 20 to 38 years (10). Conventional medical tests revealed nocturnal complex partial seizures in two of the women and night terrors in the third. It is important to recognize that seizures have long been poorly understood and accepted in Nigerian culture; such a lack of understanding may also be common in other less developed countries.

TRADITIONAL CULTURAL TREATMENTS FOR SLEEP DISORDERS

This section provides an outline of select traditional remedies for sleep problems that are used by various cultural groups drawing on their own specific beliefs or knowledge (Table 2). Because struggling to fall asleep is a common problem within many cultures, many different techniques have been sought to assist with insomnia. Folk remedies have been developed to provide relief from nightmares, excessive daytime sleepiness, and other sleep disturbances (Tables 3–5). Some of the

Table 2 Traditional remedies and products used for insomnia

Cultural origin	Name		Use
	Common	Latin	
Balkans	Buttermilk		Beverage used to aid digestion and induce sleep
Europe	Chamomile	*Chamaemelum nobile, Matricaria recutita*	Tea brewed from dried leaves is used as a sedative, an anxiolytic, and a digestive aid
Europe, Asia	Valerian; garden heliotrope	*Valeriana officinalis*	Dried roots are ground into a powder for sedative and anxiolytic purposes
Europe (Roma or Gypsy)	Lettuce	*Lactuca sativa*	Leaves are boiled for tea or dried and smoked to induce sound sleep and to alleviate constipation and anxiety
India	Basil	*Ocimum basilicum*	Tea brewed from leaves is used as a sedative
Mediterranean	Lavender	*Lavandula angustifolia*	Tea brewed from dried flowers is used as a sedative and to alleviate menstrual cramps
Mediterranean	Thyme	*Thymus vulgaris*	Tea brewed from leaves is used to induce sleep and prevent nightmares
Mexico	Citrus	*Citrus* spp	Flowers are used fresh or dried for tea to relieve tension and induce sleep
Southern Europe, Africa, Asia	Citronella grass; lemongrass	*Cymbopogon citratus, Cymbopogon nardus*	Tea brewed from tops and leaves is used as a hypnotic and to stimulate appetite, relieve menstrual cramps, and alleviate gastrointestinal complaints
Southern Europe, Mediterranean, Mexico	Lemon balm	*Melissa officinalis*	Same as above for citronella grass

(Continued)

Table 2   Traditional remedies and products used for insomnia (*Continued*)

Cultural origin	Name		Use
	Common	Latin	
Europe, eastern North America, Mexico	Linden tree	*Tilia* spp	Tea brewed from flowers is used as a tranquilizer and a hypnotic
North America (Native American), Mexico	Passion flower; maypop	*Passiflora incarnata*	Tea brewed from stems and leaves is used as a sedative and a hypnotic to alleviate insomnia, headaches, and gastrointestinal complaints
Southeast Asia	Bitter orange	*Citrus aurantium*	Dried leaves or the more potent dried peel and flowers are used to make tea for insomnia, as a calming agent, to aid digestion, and to reduce palpitations; if used in excess, it can be toxic and has been linked to heart attacks and strokes
Southeast Asia	Ginseng	*Panax* spp	Dried roots are used to make various products, such as tea, for insomnia and many other conditions
Southeast Asia	Nutmeg	*Myristica fragrans*	Dried seeds are ground and added to various beverages and foods to aid sleep
Southeast Asia	Star anise	*Illicium verum, Pimpinella anisum, Anis estrella*	Tea from dried seeds is used to aid sleep and calm nerves; the FDA has warned of toxicity in teas made from Japanese star anise (*Illicium religiosum*)
South Pacific	Kava kava	*Piper methysticum*	Roots are dried and ground into a powder or are used fresh to prepare extracts or make beverages for use as hypnotics, anxiolytics, and sleep medicines; associated with liver damage, including hepatitis and nephrotoxicity

Abbreviation: FDA, US Food and Drug Administration.

Table 3   Folk remedies and products used to induce dreams or alleviate nightmares

Cultural origin	Name		Use
	Common	Latin	
Asia	Mugwort	*Artemisia* spp	Dried leaves are stuffed into pillows to induce dreams of the future
Mediterranean	Thyme	*Thymus vulgaris*	Tea brewed from dried leaves is used to induce sleep and prevent nightmares

Table 4   Traditional remedies and products used as stimulants

Cultural origin	Name		Use
	Common	Latin	
Amazon	Guarana	*Paullina cupana*	Dried seeds (berries) are ground for tea and other beverages for use as a stimulant and to treat headache
Ethiopia	Coffee	*Coffea* spp	Dried seeds (beans) are ground for beverages or are chewed to release caffeine, which acts as a stimulant
India, China, Asia	Tea	*Camellia sinensis*	Dried leaves are brewed for tea, which contains caffeine that acts as a stimulant
Latin America	Cacao	*Theobroma cacao*	Dried seeds (beans) are ground for beverages, which contain the stimulant caffeine, and for numerous other uses
Southeast Asia	Betel palm	*Areca catechu*	Dried seeds (nuts) and leaves are ground into a powder for use in tea or as a mild stimulant
Mediterranean, Asia	Mint		Leaves are brewed for tea, which acts as a mild stimulant
	Spearmint	*Mentha spicata*	
	Peppermint	*Mentha piperita*	
West Africa	Kola tree	*Cola* spp	Dried seeds (nuts) are ground for beverages or chewed to release the stimulant caffeine, which acts as a cognitive aid

Table 5   Folk remedies and products used for other sleep-related problems

Cultural origin	Name		Use
	Common	Latin	
North America	Corn silk; maize	*Zea mays*	Strands of corn silk are boiled to make a tea to relieve water retention; it is given in the morning to children with nocturia
Northern Europe, Asia	Stinging nettle	*Urtica dioica*	Leaves are brewed for tea to use to alleviate bed-wetting

Table 6 Gemstones worn to prevent sleep problems

Cultural origin	Gemstone	Purpose
Europe in the Middle Ages	Aquamarine	To grant freedom from insomnia and to cure laziness
India (ayurvedic medicine)	Opal	To enhance prophetic dreams and reduce stress
Roman Empire	Citrine	To ensure a good night's sleep, chase away nightmares, and provide energy; worn into battle by Roman soldiers during Augustus Caesar's time
Roman Empire and ancient Egyptian civilization	Carnelian	Carved into different shapes, it is used to increase energy

Table 7 Traditional remedies used for sleep that are now controlled or illegal substances because of deleterious psychoactive properties

Cultural origin	Name		Use
	Common	Latin	
Central Asia	Cannabis, marijuana, hemp, and hashish	*Cannabis* spp	Dried leaves, flowers, and seeds are smoked or brewed to make tea or other beverages for use as a mild stimulant; oil extracted by solvents is smoked, added to food, or vaporized and inhaled
Central Europe, Asia	Opium poppy	*Papaver somniferum, P. album*	The milky exudate of unripe capsules (seed pods) is air dried to be smoked; as an insomnia treatment, it was used as early as AD 161-180 by the Roman Emperor Marcus Aurelius
East Africa, Arabia	Qat or khat	*Catha edulis*	Leaves are brewed to make tea or are chewed to release cathinone (similar to amphetamine), which acts as a stimulant
Near East (viticulture started 6000–4000 BC)	Alcohol (distilled from multiple products, including corn, rye, and barley)		Various grains are distilled to make beverages that act as intoxicants in low doses or as sedatives in higher doses
North America	Peyote cactus, mescal	*Lophophora williamsii*	The crown of the cactus, which contains mescaline that acts as a stimulant, is dried and chewed or brewed
South America	Coca	*Erythroxylon coca*	The leaves are dried and chewed, smoked, or brewed to make a beverage; all act as a stimulant

strategies used to modulate sleep or sleepiness have eventually been deemed illegal (Tables 6 and 7). Caffeine became a particularly central part of social events in the Middle East, which led to the development of elaborate serving pieces (Figure 14). In the case of opium and its derivatives, intricate vessels were crafted for the purpose of storing these highly prized substances (Figure 15).

Insomnia is among the top 10 conditions for which people in the United States most frequently use complementary and alternative medicine (Figure 16). The most common alternative therapy for any condition is prayer for one's own health (43% of U.S. adults), having others pray for one's health (24%), and using a prayer group (10%) (National Center for Health Statistics 2004) (11). Praying for another person's benefit (i.e., intercessory prayer) is most widely used for patients with life-threatening diseases such as cancer. However, an Internet search for "prayer" as an intervention for "insomnia" or "sleeplessness" will yield multiple references and requests for intercessory prayer for persons with subacute and chronic insomnia. The frequency with which prayer is used as the primary means to alleviate insomnia is unknown. Some patients describe prayer as a relaxation technique they use to reduce tension and facilitate sleep. Prayers for alleviation of insomnia and nightmares are mentioned in the *Medicine of the Prophet* by As-Suyuti (12). Praying in Islam demands periods of inaction intermingled with different positions (e.g., standing, bowing, and prostrating), which leads to relaxation of both the body and the mind (Figure 17).

Within the tradition of the Catholic church, prayers to ask for help with insomnia could be directed before the reforms of the 1960s to a group of Christian saints called "the seven sleepers of Ephesus" (Figure 18) (13). The story dates from around AD 250 when seven young men accused of being Christians sought sanctuary in a mountain cave. While praying, they fell asleep. The Roman Emperor Decius ordered that the cave be sealed with them inside. The men, who were supposedly discovered and awakened by a farmer about 150 years later, believed that they had slept for only 1 night. However, during the intervening years, Christianity had spread across the region near Ephesus. This myth was embraced within the Christian church of the Byzantine era and a similar story was incorporated into the *Koran* (14).

Many cultural practices promote a relaxed state and have been used to prevent or manage sleeplessness. Ancient Egyptians and Greeks, including Aristotle and Hippocrates, believed that spirits in the brain could cause arousal. Navajo Indians in the southwestern U.S. continue to seek care for insomnia from native healers who practice elaborate rituals to help ill persons regain balance and recover their health (15).

In ayurvedic medicine, precious and semiprecious gems are believed to interact with the vedic astrologic system (Table 6). They relate to specific planets and produce a balancing effect that moderates human disease.

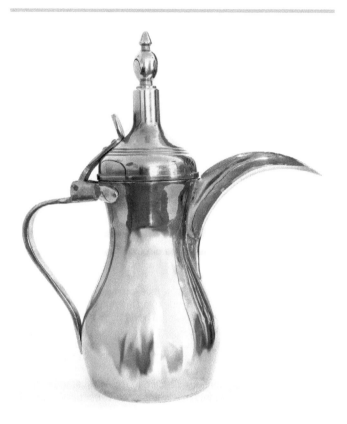

Figure 14 The ornate coffeepots used in Middle Eastern cultures illustrates the importance of the ritual of making and serving coffee. Arabian coffeepot. (Photograph from Paul Cowan. [Used with permission.])

Rituals and Symbolic Objects to Cure Sleep Complaints

To cure the conditions of susto or espanto found in Mexican-American culture, both of which are associated with insomnia, Mexican traditional folk healers called *curanderos* typically combine into several rituals some of the elements of Catholicism with herbal remedies. One cure consists of a series of rituals performed over three consecutive nights. The patient lies supine on the bed with his arms outstretched like a cross. His body is "rinsed" with an alum rock or a whole egg rubbed over the skin, then swept with a broom of herbs, typically made from horehound, rosemary, California peppertree, redbrush, or naked-seed weed. A variant of this practice calls for the curandero to bless the afflicted person's bed with a brush made of cenizo and to use holy water to cleanse and bless the person. The folk healer recites prayers from his personal prayer book and the Christian Apostles' Creed, after which the patient's spirit is called upon to return. The herb brush is later arranged in the shape of a cross and placed under the patient's pillow. Sometimes pomegranate leaves are also used in these ceremonies (8).

In modern Africa, for patients affected by ogun oru, traditional folk healers sometimes work side by side with Christian clergy. Both groups use spiritual practices to fend off the spiritual attack. Some healers and clergy believe that afflicted women are being punished by a "spirit husband" for their loyalty to their earthly husbands. Others believe that ogun oru results from women being fed toxic food produced as a result of witchcraft directed at them. The traditional healer

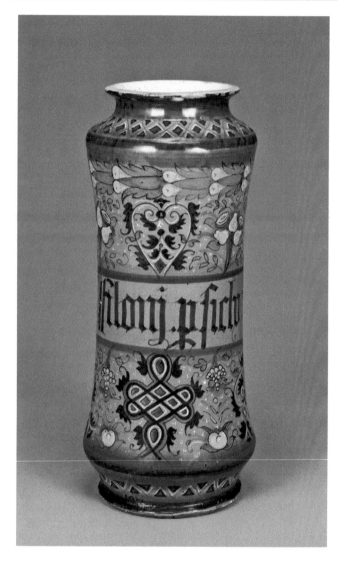

Figure 15 Tin-glazed earthenware (circa 1520-1530) used as a pharmacy vessel for "Persian philonium" made from ingredients such as opium, saffron, white pepper, pearls, and amber. (From The J. Paul Getty Museum, Los Angeles. [Used with permission.])

might call for a sacrifice to appease the witches. Spiritual intervention involves fasting, praying, nighttime vigils, and rituals of spiritual deliverance involving food, red or white candles, cloth, spiritual perfume, coconuts, and a whole egg. When traditional methods prove unsuccessful, the patients may be referred for conventional medical assessment and treatment, including anticonvulsant medication (10).

For more than 5,000 years, yoga has been used in India to promote health as a component of ayurvedic medicine. The basic tenet is to restore harmony and cure illness by maintaining the balance of the three doshas (vata, pitta, and kapha) and the elements they represent. Treatment involves eliminating impurities through cleansing rituals such as the use of enemas, by fasting, and by adhering to special diets. Symptoms are reduced by practicing yoga exercises, stretching, breathing, meditating, and lying in the sun. As a relaxation technique, yoga combines movement and meditation to minimize worry

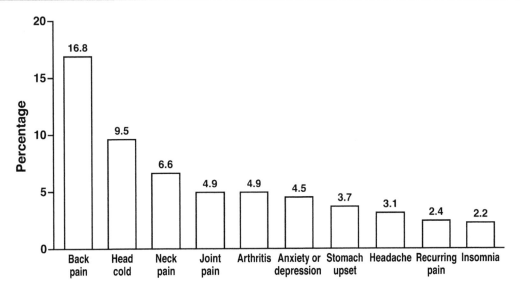

Figure 16 Insomnia is among the diseases and conditions for which complementary and alternative therapy (excluding the use of megavitamins and prayer) is most commonly used. (From National Center for Complementary and Alternative Medicine, National Institutes of Health, Bethesda, MD, 2004.)

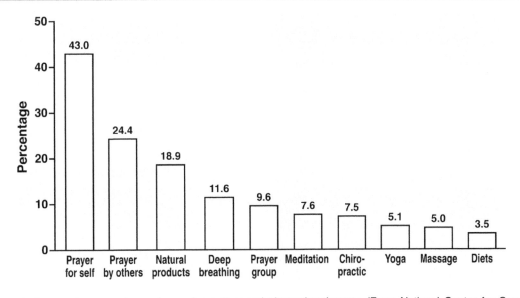

Figure 17 Prayer is the most commonly used complementary and alternative therapy. (From National Center for Complementary and Alternative Medicine, National Institutes of Health, Bethesda, MD, 2004.)

and anxiety. As worry is reduced, harmony is increased. Massage or vital points therapy using the 107 targets where energy is stored can be used to reduce pain and decrease fatigue. Herbs, plant products, oils, spices, and other substances are used, often in combination, to heal, promote vitality, or relieve pain. However, some of these compounds have been found to contain unacceptable levels of toxic substances such as heavy metals, including lead.

Traditional Chinese medicine is based on the ancient Chinese philosophy of Tao, which stresses a balance in life between the concepts of *yin* (i.e., female: cold and passive activity) and *yang* (i.e., male: hot and active). In healthy persons, the blood and life energy called *chi* flows unobstructed along the body's 12 meridians that connect the major organs. If the flow of chi is disrupted, herbs, massage, acupuncture, and other means can be used to improve it (Figure 19).

A diverse set of beliefs and practices may influence the patient with a sleep complaint. This overview of the topic should encourage clinicians to begin to pursue possible cultural aspects of sleep problems with their patients. Asking patients why they believe that they have a particular issue and what remedies they have already tried can be fruitful. Clinicians can gain insight into why the patients perceive themselves to have developed a problem, which allows for more effective patient education. Potential treatments can then be selected that are compatible with the individual patient's belief system. The overarching goal is to provide evidence-based medical care in a culturally competent fashion that respects patient preferences whenever possible.

REFERENCES

1. Haex B. Back and Bed: Ergonomic Aspects of Sleeping. Boca Raton: CRC Press, 2005.
2. Williams SJ. Sleep and Society: Sociological Ventures Into the (Un)known. New York: Routledge, 2005.
3. Steger B, Brunt L. Night-time and Sleep in Asia and the West: Exploring the Dark Side of Life. New York: Routledge Curzon, 2003.
4. Ken Y-N. Trains Are the Japanese's Second Bedroom. What Japan Thinks [Internet] [cited 2007 Feb 28]. Available from: http://www.whatjapanthinks.com/2005/12/07/trains-are-the japaneses-second-bedroom/.
5. Simich L, Hamilton H, Baya BK. Mental distress, economic hardship and expectations of life in Canada among Sudanese newcomers. Transcult Psychiatry 2006; 43: 418–44.
6. de Rynck P. How To Read a Painting: Lessons From the Old Masters. New York: HN Abrams, 2004. p. 306–7.
7. Choi YJ, Lee KJ. Evidence-based nursing: effects of a structured nursing program for the health promotion of Korean women with Hwa-Byung. Arch Psychiatr Nurs 2007; 21: 12–6.
8. Torres E. Healing With Herbs and Rituals: A Mexican Tradition. Albuquerque: University of New Mexico Press, 2006.
9. Law S, Kirmayer LJ. Inuit interpretations of sleep paralysis. Transcult Psychiatry 2005; 42: 93–112.
10. Aina OF, Famuyiwa OO. Ogun Oru: a traditional explanation for nocturnal neuropsychiatric disturbances among the Yoruba of Southwest Nigeria. Transcult Psychiatry 2007; 44: 44–54.
11. Mayo Clinic Book of Alternative Medicine: The New Approach to Using the Best of Natural Therapies and Conventional Medicine. New York: Time Inc Home Entertainment, 2007.
12. As-Suyuti JA. As-Suyuti's Medicine of the Prophet. London: Ta-Ha, 1994.
13. Herbermann CG, Pace EA, Pallen CB, Shahan TJ, Wayne JJ (eds). The Catholic Encyclopedia: An International Work of Reference on the Constitution, Doctrine, Discipline, and History of the Catholic Church. New York: The Encyclopedia Press, Inc, 1913.
14. Ali AY. The Qur'an: Translation. 5th ed. Elmhurst (NY): Tahrike Tarsile Qur'an, 2000. pp. 184–92.
15. Kim C, Kwok YS. Navajo use of native healers. Arch Intern Med 1998; 9: 2245–49.

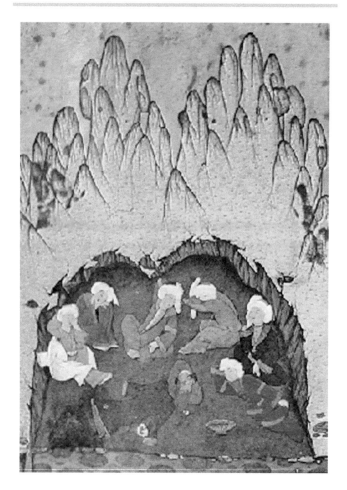

Figure 18 Turkish miniature depicting the seven sleepers of Ephesus. (From Zubat-al Tawarikh in the Museum of Turkish and Islamic Art, Istanbul, Turkey, dedicated to Sultan Murad III in 1583. [Used with permission.])

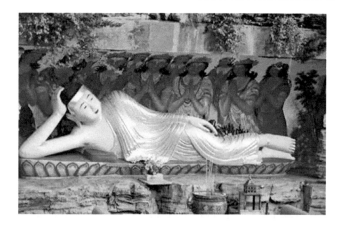

Figure 19 Statues of the sleeping Buddha are found in numerous cultures, such as those of India and Thailand. The sleep of the Buddha is viewed as an act of prayer. (From ThaiWorldView. [Used with permission.])

3

Animals and Sleep

Lois E. Krahn, MD, and Timothy I. Morgenthaler, MD

ABBREVIATIONS

EEG, electroencephalograph; electroencephalographic

NREM, non–rapid eye movement

REM, rapid eye movement

SLEEP IN ANIMALS

The American inventor Thomas A. Edison exhibited a remarkable lack of understanding in 1903 about the sleep habits of animals. His misperceptions led him to make an unfounded observation, proven eventually to be erroneous, about the omnipresence and need for sleep across the animal kingdom.

> Sleep is an acquired habit. Cells don't sleep. Fish swim about in the water all night; *they* don't sleep. Even a horse don't [sic] sleep, he just stands still and rests. A man don't [sic] need any sleep.
> (Thomas A. Edison, circa 1903) (1)

Since Edison's era, research has focused on the tremendous diversity that exists in the duration, physiology, and setting of sleep across species. These discoveries have led to insights on the role of sleep for both animals (Figure 1) and humans. Depending on the class and species of animal, intriguing differences have been detected that clarify the function and risks of sleep. Sleep research in animals is necessarily multidisciplinary and requires both tenacity and innovation.

Investigators collecting electroencephalographic (EEG) data from animals face huge technical challenges; these hurdles are even bigger for projects conducted in the wild. Animals in captivity, whether on a farm or in a zoo or laboratory, typically have sleep patterns that have adapted to their environment. Studying the sleep of animals in the wild enables the recognition of sleep patterns that have evolved to serve the needs of specific animals while they are hunting for food, avoiding predators, preserving body temperature, and maintaining buoyancy or migration.

This chapter highlights the discoveries regarding sleep physiology, sleep patterns, and sleep disorders that occur naturally in several animals. Animal models of sleep disorders have been developed specifically to facilitate research and have resulted in exciting scientific discoveries; however, an examination of these advances is beyond the scope of this chapter.

Detecting Sleep in Animals

The data needed to confirm whether an animal is asleep have generated considerable discussion. EEG data are the most definitive; however, obtaining EEG data is seldom feasible for animals not in captivity or for very small creatures (e.g., insects). When EEG leads are placed on a free-roaming animal in its natural habitat, there is always the potential for them to malfunction or to become dislodged. Accordingly, given the limited availability of EEG data for many species, there has been a clear need for consensus about which behaviors indicate sleep (Figure 2) (Table 1).

Fish, Amphibians, and Reptiles

Little is known about sleep in fish. Contrary to Thomas Edison's expectation, fish have been observed to exhibit behaviors thought to represent sleep, including periods of inactivity and decreased responsiveness to available food. Sleep has been studied in only a few of the thousands of species of fish. During periods of inactivity, for example, tilapia have been observed to be less responsive to noxious stimuli, which suggests that they are asleep (2).

No data are available regarding non–rapid eye movement (NREM) or REM (rapid eye movement) sleep in fish. Nonetheless, zebra fish, likely because of convenience and rapid reproduction, in particular are increasingly used in gene expression experiments that include efforts to better understand the role of neurochemistry in influencing sleep-wake behavior (Figure 3). However, hypocretin loss in the zebra fish is associated with insomnia and therefore appears to function basically in a fashion opposite to that in humans (3).

Amphibians represent a large class of animals that bridges the aquatic and terrestrial environments. Frogs and toads are known to have periodic inactivity suggestive of sleep, although whether it represents actual sleep or a state of drowsiness has been debated (4). However, to protect against predators, the bullfrog is believed to maintain vigilance even when inactive. To date REM sleep has not been identified in amphibians.

Birds

The sleep of birds is fairly similar to that of humans and can be subdivided into three main states: 1) active sleep, 2) quiet sleep, and 3) wakefulness. Wakeful birds keep their eyes open and scan their environment. During active or REM sleep, their eyes are closed and clusters of eye movements have been recorded (5). Relaxed muscle tone leading to head drooping has been observed in geese and ducks. Avian REM sleep is bihemispheric. In contrast, quiet or NREM sleep in birds is primarily unihemispheric (5). Unihemispheric sleep has been described as occurring more often in mallard ducks sleeping in a setting with more risks for predators, which suggests that it serves to increase vigilance (Figure 4) (6).

Birds have frequent sleep-wake transitions. This has led to speculation that vigilance is increased by intermittent brief episodes of quiet sleep (7).

Sleep positions in birds are incredibly diverse, ranging from parrots that sleep hanging upside down by their feet to birds sleeping perched on a wire. Many birds sleep with the head turned so that the bill rests on the shoulders. The

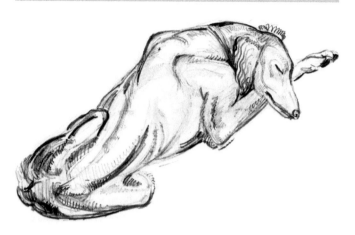

Figure 1 Typical Repose of a Sleeping Dog. A sleeping dog may curl up or stretch out in various other relaxed positions, such as with the head resting on the front paws. (Pencil drawing titled *Dog Sleeping* by American artist Paul Manship.) (From Smithsonian American Art Museum, bequest of Paul Manship. [Used with permission.])

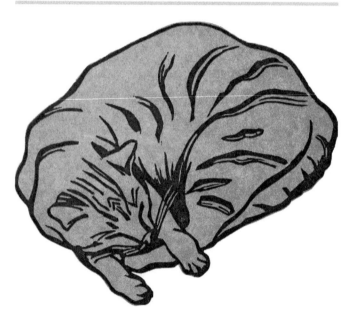

Figure 2 Typical Repose of a Sleeping Cat. Cats usually curl up in a tight ball to sleep. (Color linoleum cut titled *Chrissie* by Rowland Lyon.) (From Smithsonian American Art Museum, gift of the artist. [Used with permission.])

Table 1 Animal behaviors that indicate sleep

Selects a particular site to sleep
Adopts a specific posture
Assumes a quiet relaxed state
Passes rapidly from wakefulness to sleep
Awakens with difficulty
Develops rebound sleepiness after being sleep deprived

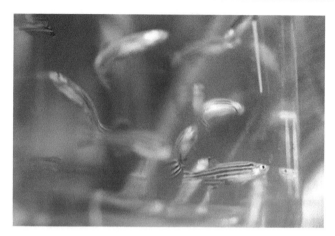

Figure 3 Motionless Zebra Fish. The zebra fish is an aquatic animal model used to study the genetics of the sleep mechanism.

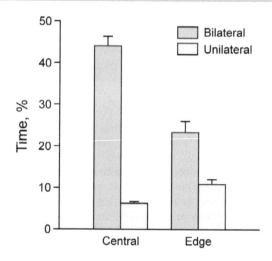

Figure 4 Percentage of Time Mallard Ducks Spend With Bilateral vs Unilateral Eye Closure. Electroencephalographic data averaged for 16 ducks show that ducks sleep in linear groups of 4 birds, with 2 in the central position (left) and 2 on the periphery or edge (right) of the group. Those in the central position have more bilateral eye closure, whereas those on the edge have more unilateral eye closure. (From Rattenborg et al. [6] [Used with permission.])

European swift has been documented with radar as having the capacity during migration to sleep while flying with the necessary muscle activity controlled by spinal reflexes (8).

Mammals

The sleep of mammals has been investigated more extensively than has the sleep of other animals with the recognition that great variability exists. For other classes of animals, confirming sleep in a particular animal, especially in a natural setting, is quite challenging. Sleep must be differentiated from hibernation and medical conditions such as coma. Sleep is presumed to occur when the mammal is observed awakening promptly from apparent somnolence. When available, polysomnographic recordings or characteristic EEG waves can be used to confirm the presence of sleep, but these data are rarely available for wild animals.

Newborn mammals have more REM sleep than adults, and the percentage of REM sleep declines as the brain matures (9). Physiological variations in REM sleep, most notably the lack of complete muscle paralysis, exists in some species. The lack of complete muscle paralysis in a sleeping dog can lead to twitching, pawing, sniffing, whimpering, and even barking. These sleep movements are considered to be physiological rather than representative of a pathologic condition because they are ubiquitous in dogs and typically do not lead to adverse consequences. These canine sleep behaviors undoubtedly exist on a continuum with the human disorder parasomnia REM sleep behavior disorder, which involves abnormal behaviors during REM sleep that can result in potentially dangerous actions, including flailing of the arms, kicking, and shouting. This disorder primarily affects aging men with degenerative neurological disorders (10). Canines that merit treatment because of injurious behavior have been responsive to clonazepam, the same medication used for parasomnias in humans. These behaviors have been theorized to be an enactment of the dog's dreams, although there is no way to confirm the existence of dreams in dogs or in any other nonhuman creature. These movements were sufficiently well known by the middle of the 20th century to have been incorporated into the Walt Disney animated films *Cinderella* in 1950 and *Lady and the Tramp* in 1955 (11).

Aquatic mammals live in an environment where the sustained inactivity associated with sleep places the animals at risk of drowning. Two groups of aquatic mammals have been studied, cetaceans (e.g., dolphins and beluga whales) and otariids (e.g., sea lions and fur seals) (12). The cetaceans never experience bihemispheric sleep but do sleep with one hemisphere at a time, whether swimming at depth or floating on the surface. Interestingly, bottlenose dolphins in the northern hemisphere circle counterclockwise while sleeping. The life of the seal differs because this aquatic mammal spends time ashore. The sleep of the seal while on land is bihemispheric. At sea the seal rolls to one side and keeps one eye open while using a single flipper to swim. Recordings of seals at sea have revealed only unihemispheric NREM sleep vs REM sleep or a combination. Studies of aquatic mammals have generated fundamental questions about whether the REM state and, indeed, whether sleep itself as defined by inactivity followed by abrupt reversal, are universal conditions in all animals.

The duration of sleep appears to be regulated by homeostatic and circadian factors. Longer durations are observed in carnivores, perhaps because of the greater weight of their brains or their lower metabolic rate. In contrast, the giraffe, a large herbivore that needs to graze often to meet its caloric needs, has a total sleep time of as little as two hours over a 24-hour period (9). It has long been believed that the sloth, an animal so sedentary that algae sometimes grows on its fur, sleeps more than any other mammal, with a sleep time ranging from 15 to 20 hours a day (13). Newer reports based on EEG results rather than on behavioral data have revealed that the sloth has a substantially lower total sleep time of 9.5 hours.

Circadian patterns of sleep and wakefulness in terrestrial mammalian species include major sleep periods that are diurnal, nocturnal, polyphasic, and irregular (Table 2). Several species, including the squirrel monkey, apes, and humans, can alternate circadian patterns from monophasic to biphasic when necessary. Studies based on physiological data collected

Table 2 Predominant sleep-wake patterns in select species

Monophasic sleep	
Nocturnal sleep	**Diurnal sleep**
Bird (most types)	Barred owl
Chimpanzee	Cockroach
Elephant	Fox
Gorilla	Kangaroo
Horse	Opossum
Human	Rat
Orangutan	Wolf
Tamarin	

Polyphasic sleep
Cat
Cow
Dog
Hedgehog
Lemur
Sheep

Unihemispheric slow-wave sleep
Armadillo
Beluga whale
Bottlenose dolphin
Fur seal (at sea)
Reptile
White whale

in the wild are needed to examine and better understand the balance of homeostatic and circadian factors influencing sleep-wake patterns.

The choice of sleep location and posture while asleep varies by species and environmental conditions. Aquatic animals must continue to maintain some degree of movement in order to keep swimming. Many terrestrial mammals find a well-defended or hidden location where they can close their eyes and sleep in a recumbent position. The *Papio* sp of baboon sleeps on its heels high up in trees, presumably sacrificing comfort to increase its safety from predators (14). Apes create a nest on the ground each night in which to sleep. Many large herbivores, including giraffes and elephants, sleep while standing, most likely to reduce their vulnerability to predators. Domesticated cattle sleep with their eyes open, presumably to watch out for anything that might threaten them (12). Horses adapt the depth of their sleep and their posture while asleep to avoid deep sleep when alone, because of the need to be vigilant for predators. Most equine sleep is obtained while standing (Figure 5). The stifle joint, a structure that presses the femur to the patella, prevents the horse's legs from bending even when its muscles are relaxed. Horses achieve REM sleep only when lying down.

Rituals that precede sleep have also been observed, although their function is unclear. One example is the instinctual action of dogs to circle their sleeping spot several times before lying down.

SLEEP DISORDERS IN MAMMALS
Narcolepsy

Narcolepsy is the best-known example of a natural model of a sleep disorder in any animal. In the 1970s, symptoms of cataplexy were reported in a French poodle that developed a transient muscle paralysis whenever it was excited by the

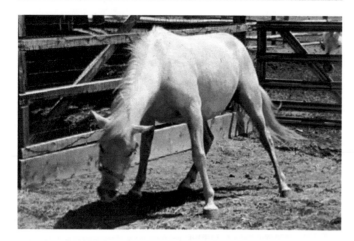

Figure 5   Horse With Narcolepsy. Compared with a typically sleeping horse, which usually stands with its eyelids partially open and its head hanging at a medium height, a horse with narcolepsy might close its eyes, hang its head nearly to hoof level, and buckle its forelimbs. (Photograph courtesy of Dwight G. Bennett, DVM, PhD, Diplomate ACT. [Used with permission.])

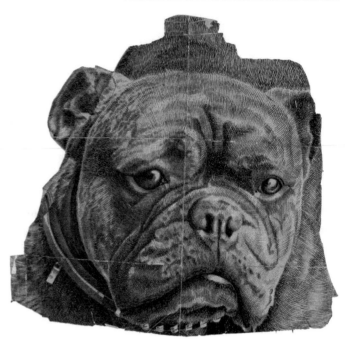

Figure 6   English Bulldog. The English bulldog is one of several breeds of dogs with brachycephalic airways that increase the risk of sleep apnea. (Ink drawing of a bulldog head, undated/Benson Bond Moore, artist, drawing: ink; 28 x 28 cm. Courtesy of the Benson Bond Moore papers, 1895-1995, Archives of American Art, Smithsonian Institution. [Used with permission.])

prospect of being given food (15). Dogs with narcolepsy also exhibit excessive daytime sleepiness and nap more than normal dogs do. Polysomnography has confirmed that the sleep in these dogs is fragmented by frequent transitions between sleep and wakefulness and by changes in REM sleep similar to those in the human form of the disease (16). Narcoleptic symptoms were subsequently found in dachshunds, beagles, collies, Doberman pinschers, and Labrador retrievers. Although the genetic transmission of narcolepsy has been determined to be sporadic in most dog breeds, narcolepsy is almost always associated with an autosomal recessive gene in Dobermans and Labradors. With great effort, researchers have developed pedigrees of affected animals for study purposes. The mechanism involves the hypocretin system with a mutation of the hypocretin receptor, type 2, in contrast to the hypocretin 1 deficiency in humans with narcolepsy (17). In extremely rare cases, dogs have been reported to lack the hypocretin 1 neuropeptide in cerebrospinal fluid, which is the same finding described in humans with narcolepsy (18). One dog was identified as having a deficiency of the ligand, thus permitting experimental trials of intravenous hypocretin 1 that led to brief reductions in its cataplexy (19).

Although cataplexy has been studied to a more limited degree than either narcolepsy or sleep, it has also been documented in numerous nonhuman mammals, including horses and sheep (16). Described in many breeds of horses, including Thoroughbreds and Arabians, cataplectic episodes last approximately a minute, with behavioral manifestations that range from buckling of the forelegs that results in falls to kneeling, staggering, sagging lips, or closing of the eyes.

Obstructive Sleep Apnea

Obstructive sleep apnea has frequently been reported in the English bulldog and in other dog breeds such as Lhasa apsos, Shih Tzus, and boxers that have brachycephalic airway syndrome (20). The American Kennel Club standards for these

canine pedigrees specify a thick neck, an upturned snout, and a pronounced jaw structure (Figure 6). Selective genetic inbreeding has produced changes in the English bulldog's facial structure that in turn have contributed to collapse of the upper airway. This breed of dog has proved to be a valuable animal model for the study of obstructive sleep apnea. English bulldogs have been used for studies of the relationship of dilating muscle activity in the upper airway and of specific sleep stages, as well as for trials of various pharmacological agents such as L-tryptophan, trazodone, and odansetron (21). Dogs requiring corrective treatment for obstructive sleep apnea may undergo upper airway surgery similar to a UPPP (uvulo-palatopharyngoplasty).

Insomnia

Normal sleep in the guinea pig has been described as a possibly naturally occurring model of insomnia (22). Polysomnography has documented that in natural conditions these rodents have reduced sleep quality with frequent sleep-wake transitions and no preference for either diurnal or nocturnal activity (23). This sleep pattern putatively allows the animal to remain more vigilant of its surroundings and presumably to be safer from predators. The guinea pig insomnia model has been proposed as a natural model for intervention. When the guinea pig is medicated with a benzodiazepine, total sleep time increases and state transitions become less frequent. The understanding of sleep and sleep disorders has increased significantly in the years since Thomas Edison published his observations. What has been learned about sleep in animals has aided the understanding of sleep mechanisms and sleep pathology in humans. As technology and funding permit, more research on sleep in animals is expected to lead to future discoveries.

REFERENCES

1. Edison in His Laboratory. Harper's Magazine. 1932 Sep: 407.
2. Shapiro CM, Hepburn HR. Sleep in a schooling fish, *Tilapia mossambica*. Physiol Behav 1976; 16: 613–5.
3. Yokogawa T, Marin W, Faraco J, et al. Characterization of sleep in zebrafish and insomnia in hypocretin receptor mutants. PLoS Biol 2007; 5: e277.
4. Hobson JA. Electrographic correlates of behavior in the frog with special reference to sleep. Electroencephalogr Clin Neurophysiol 1967; 22: 113–21.
5. Rattenborg NC, Amlaner CJ, Lima SL. Behavioral, neurophysiological and evolutionary perspectives on unihemispheric sleep. Neurosci Biobehav Rev 2000; 24: 817–42.
6. Rattenborg NC, Lima SL, Amlaner CJ. Facultative control of avian unihemispheric sleep under the risk of predation. Behav Brain Res 1999; 105: 163–72.
7. Roth TC 2nd, Lesku JA, Amlaner CJ, Lima SL. A phylogenetic analysis of the correlates of sleep in birds. J Sleep Res 2006; 15: 395–402.
8. Cramp S editor. The birds of the western paleartic. Oxford University Press, 1985. p. 661-3.
9. Siegel JM. Clues to the functions of mammalian sleep. Nature 2005; 437: 1264–71.
10. Olson EJ, Boeve BF, Silber MH. Rapid eye movement sleep behaviour disorder: demographic, clinical and laboratory findings in 93 cases. Brain 2000; 123 (Pt 2): 331–9.
11. Iranzo A, Schenck CH, Fonte J. REM sleep behavior disorder and other sleep disturbances in Disney animated films. Sleep Med 2007; 8: 531–6. Epub 2007 May 18.
12. Siegel JM. Do all animals sleep? Trends Neurosci 2008; 31: 208–13. Epub 2008 Mar 6.
13. Rattenborg NC, Voirin B, Vyssotski AL, et al. Sleeping outside the box: electroencephalographic measures of sleep in sloths inhabiting a rainforest. Biol Lett 2008; 4: 402–5.
14. Anderson JR. Sleep-related behavioural adaptations in free-ranging anthropoid primates. Sleep Med Rev 2000; 4: 355–73.
15. Delashaw JB Jr, Foutz AS, Guilleminault C, Dement WC. Cholinergic mechanisms and cataplexy in dogs. Exp Neurol 1979; 66: 745–57.
16. Nishino S, Mignot E. Pharmacological aspects of human and canine narcolepsy. Prog Neurobiol 1997; 52: 27–78.
17. Lin L, Faraco J, Li R, et al. The sleep disorder canine narcolepsy is caused by a mutation in the hypocretin (orexin) receptor 2 gene. Cell 1999; 98: 365–76.
18. Nishino S, Ripley B, Overeem S, Lammers GJ, Mignot E. Hypocretin (orexin) deficiency in human narcolepsy. Lancet 2000; 355: 39–40.
19. Nishino S. Clinical and neurobiological aspects of narcolepsy. Sleep Med 2007; 8: 373–99. Epub 2007 Apr 30.
20. Kimoff RJ, Makino H, Horner RL, et al. Canine model of obstructive sleep apnea: model description and preliminary application. J Appl Physiol 1994; 76: 1810–7.
21. Veasey SC, Fenik P, Panckeri K, Pack AI, Hendricks JC. The effects of trazodone with L-tryptophan on sleep-disordered breathing in the English bulldog. Am J Respir Crit Care Med 1999; 160(5 Pt 1): 1659–67.
22. Tobler II, Franken P, Trachsel L, Borbely AA. Models of sleep regulation in mammals. J Sleep Res 1992; 1: 125–7.
23. Gvilia I, Darchia N, Darchia TO. The guinea pig as a natural model of insomnia. Actas de Fisiologia 2001; 7: 21.

4

The Physiology of Sleep

Michael H. Silber, MBChB, FCP (SA)

ABBREVIATIONS

EEG, electroencephalogram; electroencephalography

EMG, electromyogram; electromyography

EOG, electro-oculogram; electro-oculography

GABA, γ-aminobutyric acid

NREM, non–rapid eye movement

REM, rapid eye movement

SCN, suprachiasmatic nuclei

VLPO, ventrolateral preoptic

THE STATES OF WAKE AND SLEEP

Human existence can be conceptualized as occurring in three states, one of wakefulness and two of sleep. The discovery in 1953 that periods of rapid eye movement (REM) occur during sleep (1) led to a realization that sleep consists of two states with much different physiology. Non–rapid eye movement (NREM) sleep makes up most of a person's sleep but is interspersed by periods of REM sleep. In a young adult, sleep is composed of approximately five successive cycles, each consisting of a period of NREM sleep followed by a period of REM sleep. In the early cycles of sleep, the duration of NREM sleep considerably exceeds that of REM sleep, but in the later cycles, REM sleep makes up a larger percentage of each cycle (Figure 1).

The different states of wakefulness and sleep can be most accurately described by their electrophysiological characteristics on electroencephalography (EEG), electro-oculography (EOG), and electromyography (EMG). An EEG of the state of wakefulness is characterized by alpha rhythm, which consists of 9-Hz to 10-Hz rhythmic sinusoidal waves recorded over the occipital head region during relaxed wakefulness with the eyes closed (Figure 2). NREM sleep is subdivided into three stages of increasing depth: stages N1, N2, and N3 sleep (2). In stage N1 sleep, low-amplitude, mixed-frequency (predominantly 4-Hz to 7-Hz) rhythms replace alpha activity and slow, rolling eye movements, predominantly horizontal (Figure 3), develop. The two signs of the descent into stage N2 sleep are the presence of K complexes and sleep spindles (Figure 4). K complexes are high-amplitude diphasic waves lasting at least 0.5 second; they are recorded maximally over the frontal regions. Sleep spindles are trains of 11-Hz to 16-Hz (predominantly 12-Hz to 14-Hz) waves that last at least 0.5 second; they are maximally expressed over the central head regions. Stage N3 sleep is characterized by slow waves (0.1–0.5 Hz) of high amplitude (at least 75 microvolts over the frontal regions), composing at least 20% (6 seconds) of each 30-second period,

or epoch, of sleep (Figure 5). During NREM sleep, decreases occur in heart rate, blood pressure, respiratory minute volume, skeletal muscle tone, and cerebral blood flow. Breathing becomes regular, except during the transition between wakefulness and sleep.

The physiological characteristics of REM sleep differ greatly from those of NREM sleep (Figure 6). The EOG shows bursts of irregular, conjugate rapid eye movements, whereas the EMG shows profound loss of skeletal muscle tone. Skeletal muscle activity persists only in the diaphragm, extraocular muscles, and middle ear muscles. The EEG shows desynchronized, low-amplitude, mixed-frequency activity with bursts of sawtooth waves (2-Hz to 4-Hz sharply contoured or serrated waves maximal over the central regions, often preceding clusters of rapid eye movements). Superimposed on muscle atonia are short bursts of transient muscle activity. Irregular acceleration occurs in the heart rate and the respiratory rate. Penile erection or clitoral engorgement occurs, thermal regulation becomes poikilothermic, cerebral blood flow increases, and vivid, emotionally charged dreams are experienced.

Total sleep time declines between childhood and age 60 years (3). Sleep efficiency (the percentage of time in bed spent asleep; determined by dividing the amount of time asleep by the amount of time in bed) decreases with age due to increased sleep latency (the amount of time from "lights out" until the onset of sleep) and increased wake time after sleep onset (Figure 7). A young adult spends about 25% percent of the night in REM sleep (Figure 8). In contrast, about 50% of a neonate's sleep is active sleep (the neonatal equivalent of REM sleep) and 50% is quiet sleep (the neonatal equivalent of NREM sleep). The percentage of slow-wave sleep declines from childhood through old age, whereas the percentage of REM sleep falls until about age 60 years. Concomitantly, the percentage of stages N1 and N2 sleep increase with age.

THE GENESIS OF WAKEFULNESS

Arousal and consciousness are mediated through a series of interlocking neural pathways. Two ascending systems, the cholinergic and monoaminergic pathways, are stabilized by a third regulatory system, the hypocretin (also known as orexin) pathway. Together, these networks are responsible for the perception of multimodal sensory stimuli, the sense of consciousness, and the inhibition of sleep (4).

The cholinergic system originates in neurons of the dorsal pontine tegmentum, specifically, the pedunculopontine and the lateral dorsal tegmental nuclei. Their axons project to the reticular and relay nuclei of the thalamus, thereby opening the gate that controls the transmission of incoming sensory stimuli to

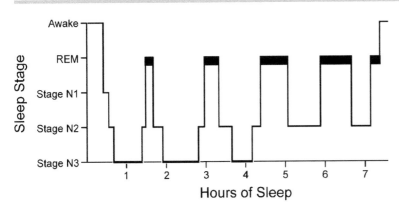

Figure 1 Normal Hypnogram in a Young Adult. This simplified representation of a hypnogram demonstrates the expected progression of a normal young adult through the stages of sleep over the course of a night. In each cycle of sleep, non–rapid eye movement sleep is followed by rapid eye movement (REM) sleep. Stage N3 (slow-wave) sleep is more evident in early cycles and REM sleep periods are longer in later cycles toward morning. Entry into REM sleep is generally through stage N2 sleep. (Adapted from Silber MH, Krahn LE, Morgenthaler TI. Sleep Medicine in Clinical Practice. New York: Taylor & Francis, 2004. [Used with permission of Mayo Foundation for Medical Education and Research.])

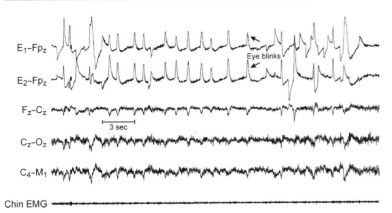

Figure 2 Stage W. This 30-second epoch of wakefulness was recorded with the subject's eyes closed. Blinking continued, visible as in-phase, upward deflections in the electro-oculogram (channels 1 and 2). The cortical electro-encephalogram shows alpha rhythm over the occipital head region (sinusoidal 9-Hz to 10-Hz activity) (channel 4). Muscle tone (measured below the chin) is relatively high (channel 6). EMG indicates electromyogram.

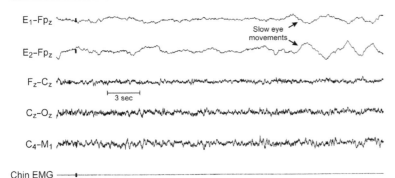

Figure 3 Stage N1 Sleep. Stage N1 sleep is the lightest stage of non–rapid eye movement sleep. Eye blinks are replaced by slow, rolling, generally horizontal eye movements, visible as out-of-phase deflections in the electro-oculogram (channels 1 and 2). Alpha rhythm is replaced by low-amplitude, mixed-frequency electroencephalogram activity, predominantly in the 4-Hz to 7-Hz range (channels 3–5). Muscle tone is reduced (channel 6). EMG indicates electromyogram.

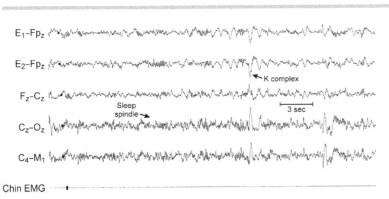

Figure 4 Stage N2 Sleep. K complexes and sleep spindles are present in stage N2 sleep. K complexes are prominent diphasic waves maximal frontally (channels 1–5) and lasting at least 0.5 second. Sleep spindles are trains of 11-Hz to 16-Hz (predominantly 12-Hz to14-Hz) activity maximal centrally (channels 4 and 5) and lasting at least 0.5 second. EMG indicates electromyogram.

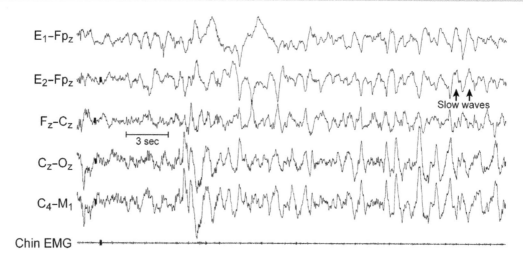

Figure 5 Stage N3 Sleep. Stage N3 sleep is characterized by high-amplitude (≥75 microvolts) slow waves (0.5 Hz) composing at least 20% of each 30-second epoch, visible in all electroencephalogram (and electro-oculogram) derivations. EMG indicates electromyogram.

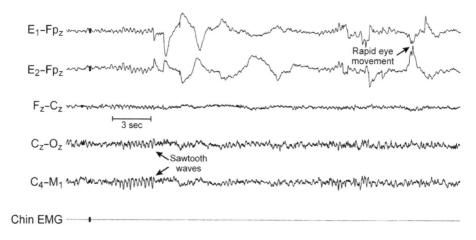

Figure 6 Stage REM Sleep. The most striking polysomnographic feature of rapid eye movement (REM) sleep is the presence of irregular, conjugate, predominantly horizontal or oblique rapid eye movements (channels 1 and 2). These out-of-phase deflections have a rapid upstroke in the first two channels and clearly differ from the blinks of wakefulness or the slow eye movements of stage N1 sleep shown in Figure 3. The electroencephalogram is desynchronized: low amplitude with mixed frequencies and lacking the rhythmicity of stages N2 and N3 sleep. A run of sawtooth waves (2-Hz to 6-Hz sharply contoured or serrated waves over the central area) often precedes REM bursts. Muscle tone is low, never higher than in any other sleep stage (channel 6). EMG indicates electromyogram.

the cerebral cortex (Figure 9) (5). Predictably, these neurons fire actively during wakefulness and are inactive during NREM sleep; paradoxically, they are also active during REM sleep (Table 1).

The monoaminergic system consists of numerous ascending axons, which are linked by the release of monoaminergic neurotransmitters (Figure 10). Neurons in the pontine locus coeruleus release norepinephrine, the pontine raphe nuclei release serotonin, the midbrain periaqueductal gray neurons release dopamine, and the hypothalamic tuberomammillary nuclei release histamine (Figure 11) (6). Stimulation of these neurons activates the cerebral cortex, thereby facilitating the processing of thalamic information (Figure 9). In addition, the neurons inhibit the primary generator of NREM sleep, the ventrolateral preoptic (VLPO) nuclei. They fire rapidly during wakefulness, discharge slowly during NREM sleep, and are inactive during REM sleep (Table 1).

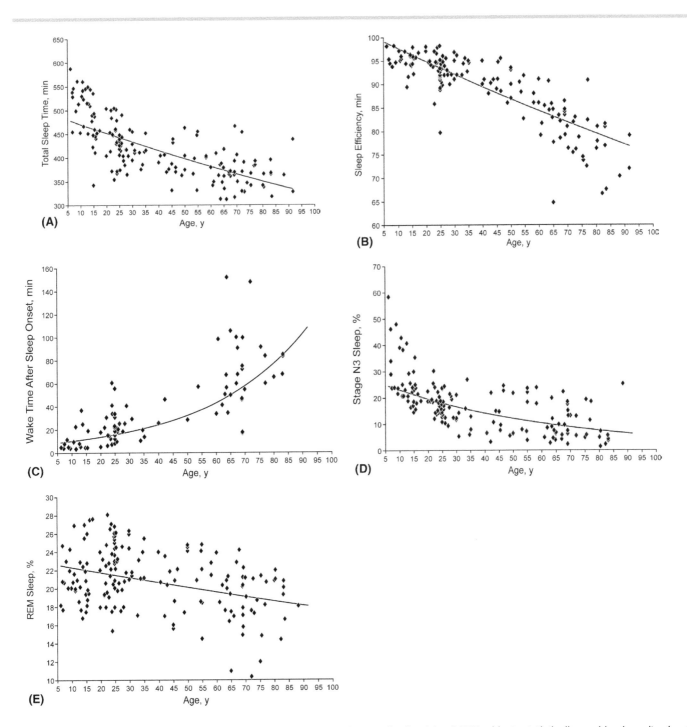

Figure 7 Changes in Sleep With Age. An extensive meta-analysis of 65 studies involving 3,577 subjects statistically combined results about changes in sleep stages with age. Despite considerable individual variability, several clear trends emerged. With increased age, there were decreases in (A) total sleep time and (B) sleep efficiency (time asleep divided by time in bed), which are accounted for by (C) increasing wake time after sleep onset. The decrease in the percentage of stage N3 sleep starts in adolescence and continues to decline throughout adulthood (D). The percentage of rapid eye movement (REM) sleep also declines with increasing age (E). Percentages of lighter non–rapid eye movement (NREM) sleep (stages N1 and N2) proportionally increase. (Adapted from Ohayon et al [3]. [Used with permission.])

The third pathway controlling arousal, the hypocretin neurons, serves as a wake-stabilizing system. The hypocretins are peptide neurotransmitters synthesized by a small cluster of cells in the posterolateral hypothalamus. Their axons, however, project widely to the cell bodies of the cholinergic and monoaminergic ascending arousal systems and to the cerebral cortex (Figure 12). They fire actively during wakefulness and are inactive during NREM and REM sleep (Table 1).

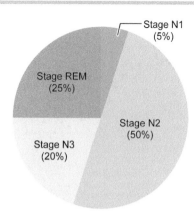

Architecture of Sleep

Figure 8 Stages of Sleep in a Healthy Young Adult. For a healthy young adult, the average percentages of the different stages of sleep summed over a night are 75% for non–rapid eye movement sleep (NREM), which encompasses stages N1, N2, and N3, and 25% for rapid eye movement sleep. Stage N2 sleep is the predominant stage of NREM sleep. (Adapted from Silber MH, Krahn LE, Morgenthaler TI. Sleep Medicine in Clinical Practice. New York: Taylor & Francis, 2004. [Used with permission of Mayo Foundation for Medical Education and Research.])

Table 1 Action of neurotransmitter systems in wakefulness and sleep

Neurons	Wakefulness	Sleep	
		NREM	REM
Cholinergic	Active	Inactive	Active
Noradrenergic	Active	Partially active	Inactive
Serotoninergic	Active	Partially active	Inactive
Hypocretinergic	Active	Inactive	Inactive

Abbreviations: NREM, non–rapid eye movement; REM, rapid eye movement.

THE GENESIS OF NREM SLEEP

The VLPO nuclei in the anterior hypothalamus are the primary generators of NREM sleep (Figure 13) (5). Releasing the inhibitory neurotransmitters γ-aminobutyric acid (GABA) and galanin, VLPO axons project to all three neuronal systems controlling arousal: the ascending cholinergic and monoaminergic neurons and the hypocretin neurons (Figure 14).

A flip-flop switch is an electronic circuit consisting of two mutually inhibitory, self-reinforcing elements. Activation of one pole of the circuit inhibits the other and thus disinhibits the first, resulting in discrete states with sharp transitions. The

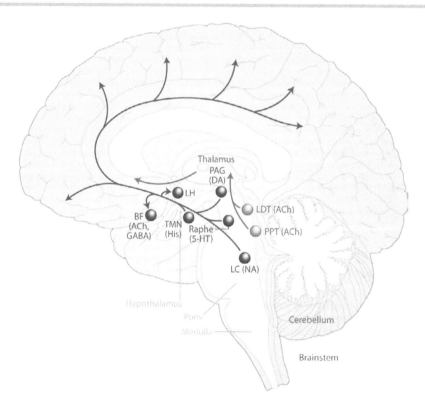

Figure 9 Monoaminergic and Cholinergic Systems: Axonal Distribution. Two ascending arousal systems maintain wakefulness. The first involves acetylcholine (ACh), a neurotransmitter with neurons in the brainstem tegmentum (pedunculopontine [PPT]) and lateral dorsal tegmental nuclei (LDT) projecting to the thalamus. The second system uses monoamine neurotransmission and is composed of several neuronal groups with different monoamine neurotransmitters. These include the locus coeruleus (LC) (norepinephrine), the raphe nuclei (serotonin [5-HT]), the periaqueductal gray (PAG) (dopamine [DA]), and the tuberomammillary nuclei (TMN) (histamine [His]). Axons from these neurons project to the cerebral cortex, the ventrolateral preoptic and basal forebrain (BF) areas, and the lateral hypothalamic (LH) areas. GABA indicates γ-aminobutyric acid; NA, noradrenaline. (Adapted from Saper et al [5]. [Used with permission.])

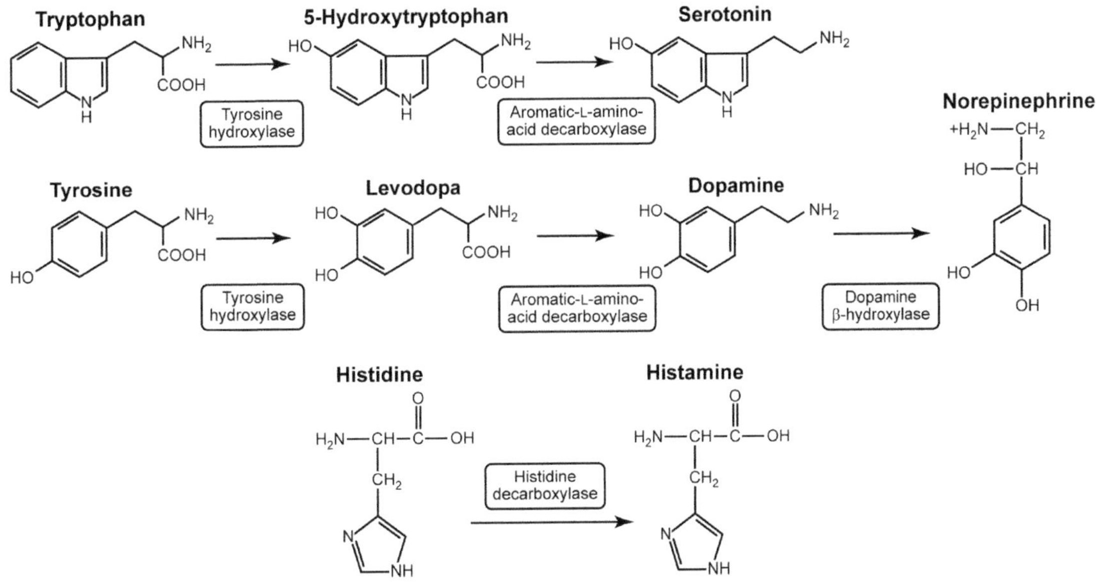

Figure 10 Monoamine Synthetic Pathways. Monoamine neurotransmission is fundamental for maintaining alertness. Knowledge of the neurochemistry of monoamine synthesis is essential for understanding many disease processes and medications used to treat sleep disorders.

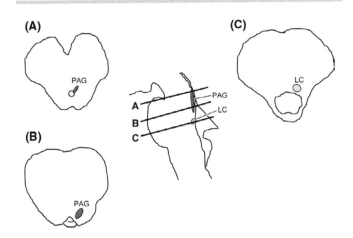

Figure 11 Monoamine Pathways. These sagittal and transverse sections through the pons and midbrain illustrate the location of (A and B), the periaqueductal gray (PAG) (dopamine-alerting system) and (C), the locus coeruleus (LC) (norepinephrine-alerting system). (Adapted from Boeve et al [6]. [Used with permission.])

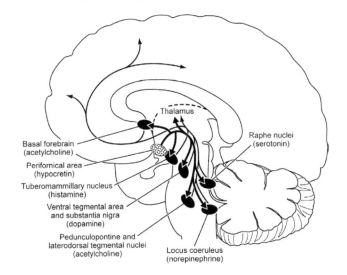

Figure 12 Hypocretin Systems: Axonal Distributions. The cells of the hypocretin (i.e., orexin) wake-stabilizing system originate in the perifornical area of the brain and their axons are widely distributed to the brainstem, hypothalamus, thalamus, basal forebrain, and cerebral cortex. (Adapted from Silber MH, Rye DB. Solving the mysteries of narcolepsy: the hypocretin story. Neurology 2001; 56: 1616–8. [Used with permission.])

weakening of either pole causes more rapid transitions between states. The monoaminergic neurons of the ascending arousal system and the neurons of the VLPO act as the two poles of a flip-flop switch (Figure 15) (5). When the monoaminergic pole fires, the VLPO is inhibited, which results in wakefulness. In contrast, when the VLPO neurons fire, the monoaminergic neurons are inhibited, which results in the onset of sleep. The switch is stabilized by the hypocretin system. During wakeful-

ness, the VLPO is inactive; thus the hypocretin-synthesizing neurons are able to discharge. Monoaminergic neurons are activated, stabilizing the state of wakefulness. During sleep, the active VLPO neurons inhibit the hypocretin neurons, which

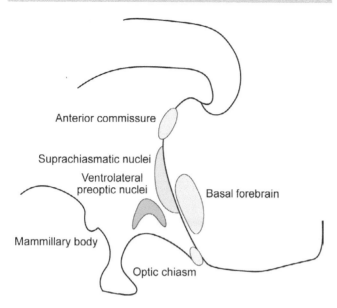

Figure 13 Nuclei of the Anterior Hypothalamus Involved in Sleep and Wakefulness. This midline sagittal view illustrates the location of the principal generator of non–rapid eye movement (NREM) sleep, the ventrolateral preoptic area in the anterior hypothalamus, and the basal forebrain, which is also involved in the generation of NREM sleep. The biological clock (i.e., the suprachiasmatic nuclei of the hypothalamus) is also shown. (Adapted from Silber MH, Krahn LE, Morgenthaler TI. Sleep Medicine in Clinical Practice. New York: Taylor & Francis, 2004. [Used with permission of Mayo Foundation for Medical Education and Research.])

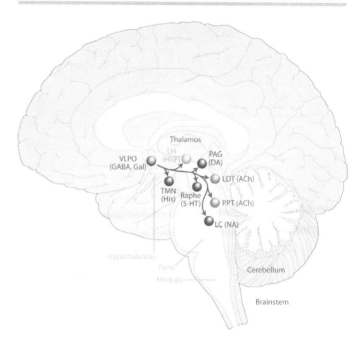

Figure 14 Ventrolateral Preoptic Axonal Distributions. Cells of the ventrolateral preoptic (VLPO) area produce the inhibitory neurotransmitters γ-aminobutyric acid (GABA) and galanin (Gal). Their axons project to the monoaminergic and cholinergic neurons of the ascending arousal systems, as well as to the cells of the lateral hypothalamus (LH) producing hypocretin (HYP). These pathways control the onset and maintenance of non–rapid eye movement sleep. ACh, acetylcholine; DA, dopamine; His, histamine; LC, locus coeruleus; 5-HT, serotonin; LDT, lateral dorsal tegmental nuclei; NA, noradrenaline; PPT, pedunculopontine; TMN, tuberomammillary nuclei; PAG, periaqueductal gray. (Adapted from Saper et al [5]. [Used with permission.])

prevent activation of the monoamine system and thus stabilize the state of NREM sleep.

NREM sleep is characterized by the intense synchronicity of neural discharges, resulting in cortical sleep spindles and high-amplitude slow waves. Sleep spindles arise in the thalamus (7) (Figure 16). Inactivity of the pontine tegmental cholinergic arousal system during NREM sleep results in hyperpolarization of GABA-releasing thalamic cells. This hyperpolarization results in the opening of calcium channels which, in turn, generate self-perpetuating action potentials at spindle frequency. The discharge of thalamocortical afferents results in similar cortical potentials that are recorded by scalp EEG as sleep spindles.

THE GENESIS OF REM SLEEP

The primary generator of REM sleep lies in the pontine tegmentum, just ventral to the locus coeruleus (8). Although this group of cells has several names, it is simplest to refer to it as the subcoeruleus region (Figure 17). Animals whose subcoeruleus regions have been ablated do not exhibit manifestations of REM sleep. During REM sleep, subcoeruleus cells fire actively ("REM-on cells") and the region demonstrates a high concentration of c-fos expression. In contrast, "REM-off cells," which are inactive during REM sleep, have been identified in the lateral pontine tegmentum and in the ventrolateral peri-

aqueductal gray matter. REM-on and REM-off cells are mutually inhibitory. The suprapontine control of REM sleep has not been fully delineated, but activation of hypothalamic cells surrounding the VLPO (extended VLPO) is known to result in inhibition of REM-off areas. This action disinhibits the neurons of the subcoeruleus region, initiating REM sleep (9) (Figure 18).

How are the diverse manifestations of REM sleep generated by a small group of pontine neurons? The pathways underlying skeletal muscle atonia are understood the best. Anterior horn cells are presynaptically inhibited by glycine or GABA-releasing neurons. In cats, glutaminergic or cholinergic neurons of the pontine tegmentum adjacent to the subcoeruleus region activate ventromedial medullary interneurons in the nucleus magnocellularis, which synapse on the anterior horn cells (8). Rats do not appear to have medullary interneurons, and pontine neurons synapse directly on inhibitory interneurons in the anterior horn (5) (Figure 19). The neural circuitry in humans is not fully known, but pontine lesions can cause REM sleep behavior disorder, a condition with loss of REM sleep atonia and resultant dream enactment behaviors, such as screaming, kicking, and punching (6).

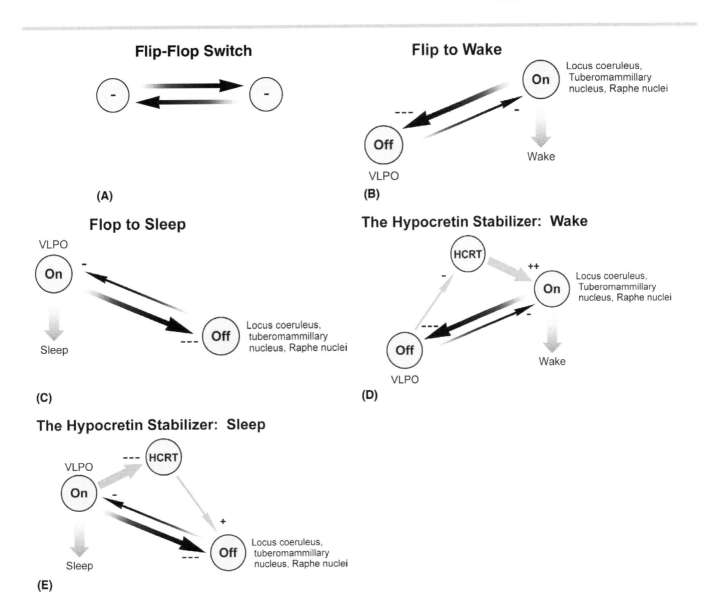

Figure 15 The Flip-Flop Switch in Wakefulness and Sleep. The principle of the flip-flop switch (A) applies to the understanding of the onset and maintenance of wakefulness (B) and sleep (C). The ventrolateral preoptic (VLPO) area and the monoaminergic arousal neurons serve as opposite poles of a flip-flop switch. The hypocretin (HCRT) system, which is active in wakefulness (D), stabilizes the wake state, whereas (E) its inhibition stabilizes sleep. Minus signs indicate inhibitory pathways; plus signs indicate excitatory pathways. The degree of inhibition or excitation is indicated by the number of signs and the thickness of the arrows. (Adapted from Saper et al [5]. [Used with permission.])

THE TIMING OF WAKE AND SLEEP

Humans sleep predominantly at night. We become drowsy by the mid-afternoon but feel more alert in the early evening. We are refreshed by short catnaps. What determines the timing of wake and sleep?

There are two sleep-control systems, homeostatic and circadian (Figure 20). The homeostatic system results in an increase in sleep drive that is directly proportional to the number of hours one spends awake. After an adequate period of sleep, the homeostatic system resets. Homeostatic control is mediated by a buildup of extracellular adenosine (4), the neuromodulator whose receptor is blocked by xanthine derivatives such as caffeine. The site of action of adenosine is uncertain; for many years, sleep-on neurons in the basal forebrain region were thought to be the target cells, but recent research has failed to confirm this hypothesis.

A complex, genetically programmed, circadian system controls the timing of most physiological processes, from hormone secretion to temperature cycles. Maximal sleepiness occurs in the late evening and at night with a second, less intense, peak in mid-afternoon. The biological clock is localized to the suprachiasmatic nuclei (SCN) of the hypothalamus (Figure 13). Genetic control is exerted by an array of circadian genes that control the synthesis of proteins, which diffuse back into the nucleus, inhibiting further gene transcription (10). This process results in molecular oscillation over an approximately circadian period.

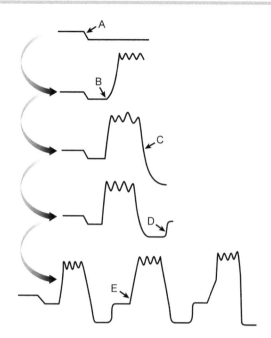

Figure 16 Genesis of Sleep Spindles. This diagram represents the membrane potential of a thalamic reticular neuron in non–rapid eye movement sleep, illustrating the genesis of sleep spindles. (A) γ-Aminobutyric acid (GABA) thalamic neurons become hyperpolarized as a result of the cessation of cholinergic input from the brainstem. (B) This hyperpolarization results in the firing of a calcium spike with a superimposed burst of action potentials. (C) The entry of calcium into the neuron is accompanied by the efflux of potassium, resulting in pronounced hyperpolarization. (D) Slight rebound depolarization occurs, which (E) again triggers a subsequent calcium spike. Thalamocortical afferent transmission results in similar changes in cortical neurons that are recorded as sleep spindles.

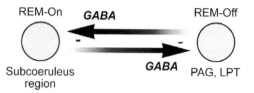

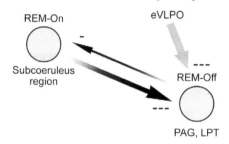

Figure 18 Control of Rapid Eye Movement (REM) Sleep. (A) A flip-flop switch is the proposed mechanism for the control of transitions between non–rapid eye movement (NREM) and REM sleep. REM-on cells in the subcoeruleus region form one pole of the switch, whereas REM-off cells in the periaqueductal gray (PAG) matter and the lateral pontine tegmentum (LPT) form the other pole. GABA indicates γ-aminobutyric acid. (B) The extended ventrolateral preoptic area (eVLPO) is active during REM sleep, inhibiting REM-off cells. This inhibition in turn results in disinhibition of the REM-on cells and the onset of REM sleep. Minus signs indicate inhibitory pathways. The degree of inhibition is indicated by the number of signs and the thickness of arrows. (Adapted from Lu et al [9]. [Used with permission.])

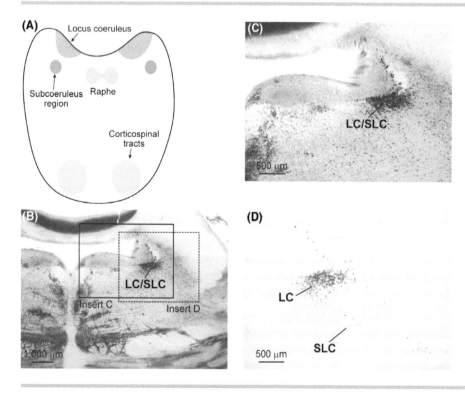

Figure 17 Localization of the Rapid Eye Movement Sleep Generator. (A) This schematic cross-section through the pons illustrates the location of the principal rapid eye movement sleep generator, the subcoeruleus region. (Adapted from Silber MH, Krahn LE, Morgenthaler TI. Sleep Medicine in Clinical Practice. New York: Taylor & Francis, 2004. [Used with permission of Mayo Foundation for Medical Education and Research.]) (B-D) A brainstem cut at the lower pons in a human subject (stained for lipofuscin [with aldehyde fuchsin] and for Nissl substance [with Darrow red]) illustrates the locus coeruleus (LC) and the subcoeruleus region (SLC) at increasing magnification. (Adapted from Boeve et al [6]. [Used with permission.])

Feline Model

Murine Model

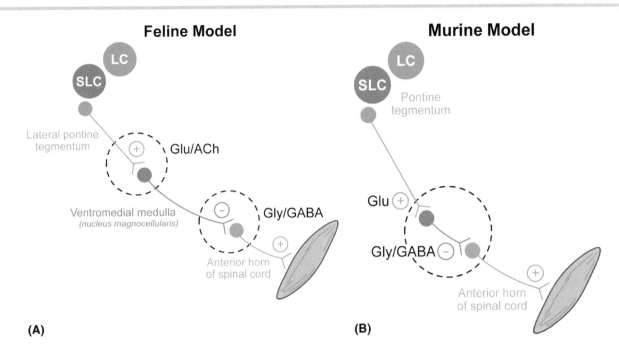

(A)

(B)

Figure 19 REM Atonia Pathways. Rapid eye movement (REM) sleep atonia is mediated through a descending inhibitory pathway from the pontine tegmentum to the alpha motor neurons in the anterior horn of the spinal cord. (A) In cats a relay station is present in the medulla, whereas (B) in rats the interneuron appears to be located in the spinal cord itself. The first-order descending neuron has glutamate (Glu) or acetylcholine (ACh) as a neurotransmitter, whereas the second-order neuron utilizes the inhibitory neurotransmitters glycine (Gly) or γ-aminobutyric acid (GABA). LC indicates locus coeruleus; SLC, subcoeruleus region.

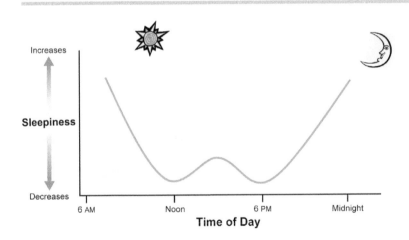

Figure 20 Homeostatic Drive and Circadian Rhythm. The timing of sleep and wakefulness depends on an interaction of homeostatic and circadian factors. The homeostatic drive (light blue) increases sleepiness from the time of waking in the morning until it is relieved by sleep at night. The circadian rhythm (dark blue) shows a minor peak of sleepiness in the early afternoon and a major peak in the evening and night.

In a constant low-illumination environment, the intrinsic periodicity of the human clock is 24.3 hours (11) (Figure 21). The influence of light during the day entrains this free-running cycle to a geophysical time of 24 hours. A special class of retinal ganglion cells secretes the pigment melanopsin, which is responsible for the transduction of short wavelength (predominantly blue) light (12). The resultant neural pathway along the retino-hypothalamic tract terminates on the SCN and alters the periodicity of its neuronal discharges. Light administered at specific times during the circadian cycle can have profound effects on circadian rhythms, delaying or advancing them, depending on the timing of the light exposure (Figure 22).

The SCN cells fire during the day and are inactive at night. The SCN outflow tract leads to the dorsomedial hypothalamic nuclei (13) (Figure 23). Axons from these neurons inhibit the VLPO and stimulate the hypocretin-synthesizing cells in the lateral hypothalamus, which results in the transition from the sleep state to the wake state. Under the control of the SCN, the pineal gland secretes the peptide hormone melatonin at night. The presence of melatonin receptors in the SCN supports the hypothesis that melatonin modulates control of circadian rhythms (Figure 24).

Ontogenic and cultural factors also play a role in the timing of sleep. Neonates sleep in many short stretches spread

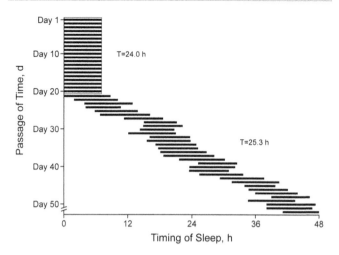

Figure 21 Temporal Isolation Experiment. In a classic temporal isolation experiment, the subject was aware of the time of the day and slept approximately 7 hours a night with regular sleep and wake times for the first 20 days (boxed horizontal bars). Then on day 21, the subject was placed in a time isolation environment with no cues to the time of day. His sleep time shifted later each day by a mean of 1.3 hours, demonstrating that the intrinsic periodicity of the human biological clock is longer than 24 hours. More recent experiments conducted in constant low illumination have shown that the true periodicity is about 24.3 hours (11). Zero on the horizontal axis represents the subject's habitual bedtime. T indicates tau, the endogenous circadian periodicity. (Adapted from Czeisler CA, Richardson GS, Coleman RM, et al. Chronotherapy: resetting the circadian clocks of patients with delayed sleep phase insomnia. Sleep 1981; 4: 1–21. [Used with permission.])

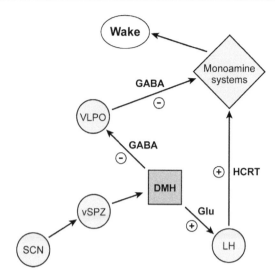

Figure 23 Outflow Pathways from the Biological Clock. The suprachiasmatic nuclei (SCN) control a vast array of circadian physiological processes. This schematic illustrates the outflow pathways from the SCN, concentrating specifically on circadian control of sleep and wakefulness. Relay neurons in the ventral subparaventricular zone of the hypothalamus (vSPZ) project to the dorsomedial nucleus of the hypothalamus (DMH) during the circadian day. Excitatory glutaminergic (Glu) neurons from the DMH project to cells in the lateral hypothalamus (LH) that produce hypocretin (HCRT), whereas GABAergic (γ-aminobutyric acid–mediated) inhibitory neurons from the DMH project to the ventrolateral preoptic (VLPO) nuclei. The inhibition of the VLPO and the conjoint release of hypocretin activate monoamine pathways, resulting in wakefulness.

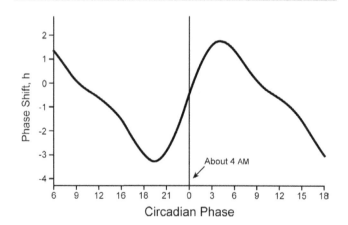

Figure 22 Human Phase Light Response Curve. Light is the most potent extrinsic factor controlling circadian timing. Light has a variable effect at different times of the circadian cycle, with early morning light shifting circadian rhythms in a backward direction ("phase advance") and late evening light resulting in a forward shift ("phase delay"). Thus a patient with delayed sleep phase disorder who can only initiate sleep at 2 AM would benefit from early morning light, whereas a patient with advanced sleep phase disorder who sleeps from 8 PM to 3 AM can be effectively treated with evening light. Circadian zero (about 4 AM), when the effects of light shift from delaying to advancing, is indicated by the vertical line.

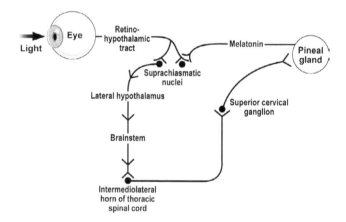

Figure 24 Melatonin Pathways. Light-induced stimulation of the suprachiasmatic nuclei results in activation of the descending sympathetic pathways through the brainstem, cervical spinal cord, and superior cervical ganglion in the neck. This results in inhibition of melatonin secretion from the pineal gland. Conversely, melatonin secretion increases in darkness. Melatonin receptors are present in the cells of the suprachiasmatic nuclei, completing a modulating feedback loop. (Adapted from Silber MH, Krahn LE, Morgenthaler TI. Sleep Medicine in Clinical Practice. New York: Taylor & Francis, 2004. [Used with permission of Mayo Foundation for Medical Education and Research.])

evenly throughout the day and night. First-decade children tend to go to bed earlier and rise earlier than adults. In mid-adolescence, a biological change occurs with the development of evening alertness and a forward shift of several hours for desired sleep and wake times. By the early to middle part of the third decade, this delayed sleep-phase pattern usually reverts to a conventional adult pattern. Some older persons may develop an advanced sleep-phase pattern, struggling to remain awake during the early evening and then waking at an undesirably early hour. Persons in cultures that embrace the siesta have developed a split pattern of sleep, with a short period of sleep occurring during the afternoon circadian dip and a longer period occurring during the night, often with a relatively late time of sleep onset. In the Middle Ages, the absence of reliable artificial light resulted in an early to bed time soon after sunset, a period of quiet wakefulness at midnight or later that lasted an hour or longer, and a second period of sleep until sunrise (14).

THE FUNCTIONS OF SLEEP

All mammals and birds sleep, as probably do other vertebrates, whereas invertebrates experience observable quiescent states similar to sleep. Clearly, this highly conserved function must play an important biological role but the identification of that role has proven elusive. Many hypotheses about the function of sleep have been proposed, and all may be partially correct. Possible functions include body repair, brain restoration, memory and learning, unlearning, immunocompetence, and thermoregulation and energy conservation.

It has been hypothesized that sleep, especially NREM sleep, is necessary for protein synthesis and for cell division and growth, thus allowing for repair of the body or restoration of brain function. REM sleep can enhance the consolidation of memory, and it may serve a role in deleting unnecessary memory traces. Sleep may help maintain immunocompetence. It may be required to maintain a positive energy balance by providing a period of rest and low metabolic activity. At the cellular or molecular level, the functions of sleep remain undetermined.

LOSS OF SLEEP

The consequences of sleep deprivation in animals and humans have interested researchers for more than a century. A series of elegant experiments conducted by Allan Rechtschaffen at the University of Chicago in the 1980s conclusively demonstrated the effects of sleep deprivation in the rat (15) (Figure 25). Sleep-deprived rats died after a mean of 21 days, with death preceded by loss of weight, ulcerative skin lesions, hypothermia, and hypercatabolism. When sleep deprivation was terminated before death, most of the rats survived, with recovery sleep characterized by large quantities of paradoxical (REM) sleep. Selective deprivation of REM sleep produced similar results, but with longer survival (mean, 37 days). Autopsy studies did not yield a definite cause of death, although subsequent unconfirmed experiments suggested that death may have resulted from septicemia.

Sustained total sleep deprivation in humans is difficult to produce experimentally. Short periods of sleep start intruding, and experiments usually terminate after a maximum of 5 to 10 days. The principal effect of such sleep deprivation is an intense desire for sleep. Psychomotor test performance

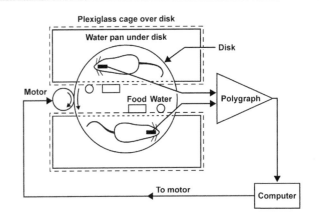

Figure 25 Sleep Deprivation in Rats. In an experimental model to study sleep deprivation in rats, the experimental and control rats are placed on a disk that can rotate over shallow pans of warm water. When the electroencephalogram of the experimental animal detects sleep, the turntable rotates and both rats have to walk in the opposite direction of the turntable's rotation to avoid falling into the water. When the control rat sleeps, the turntable does not move. This results in a 72% loss of sleep in the experimental rat but only a 9% loss in the control rat. (Adapted from Bergmann BM, Kushida CA, Everson CA, Gilliland MA, Obermeyer W, Rechtschaffen A. Sleep deprivation in the rat. II. Methodology. Sleep 1989; 12: 5–12. [Used with permission.])

declines, mood changes develop, and visual distortions or hallucinations may occur. Partial sleep deprivation of as little as two hours of sleep per night results in measurable increases in sleepiness. With increasing duration of chronic reduced sleep time, cognitive and psychomotor skills become impaired, and feelings of anxiety, sadness, and hostility may develop. Cognitive functioning progressively worsens, with little evidence for adaptation, at least over 14 days, while subjects perceive that they have overcome their initial sleepiness (16) (Figure 26). This dichotomy between objective performance measures and subjective perception of competence may result in potentially dangerous outcomes, especially in activities and occupations that may compromise public safety.

The quantity of sleep needed for recuperation after complete or partial sleep deprivation is less than the amount of sleep debt incurred. Subjects usually will sleep 12 to 15 hours on the first recovery night, with marked rebound of slow-wave sleep and increased sleep efficiency. REM sleep rebound will occur on the second recovery night, and sleep structure will usually normalize by the third night.

SLEEP AND EATING

Sleep profoundly affects almost all organ systems, but there is increasing recognition of an intricate relation between sleep and the control of appetite. Both represent fundamental biological drives regulated by the hypothalamus. Hypocretins, the excitatory neuropeptides of hypothalamic origin, stimulate wakefulness and increase food intake. The hormone leptin, secreted by adipocytes, acts on the hypothalamus to reduce

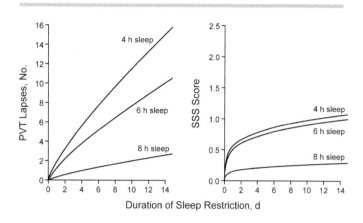

Figure 26 Effects of Partial Sleep Deprivation in Humans. In a study of partial sleep deprivation in humans, progressive difficulty with a psychomotor vigilance task (PVT) occurred with partial sleep deprivation (i.e., 4 to 6 hours of sleep per night) from baseline to 14 days, with no evidence of adaptation to the state of chronic partial sleep deprivation. In contrast, subjects did not perceive themselves as experiencing increasing sleepiness: their self-reported scores on the Stanford Sleepiness Scale (SSS) reached a plateau and did not worsen over time. Zero on x-axis indicates baseline. (Adapted from Van Dongen et al [16]. [Used with permission.])

Table 2 Characteristics of leptin and ghrelin

Characteristic	Hormone	
	Leptin	Ghrelin
Source	Adipocytes	Stomach
Target	Hypothalamus	Hypothalamus
Effect on appetite	Suppresses	Stimulates
Effect of sleep deprivation	Decreases	Increases

Table 3 The spectrum of sleep and eating disorders

Disorder	Nature of relation
Anorexia or bulimia nervosa	Eating at night
Kleine-Levin syndrome	Hypersomnia; binge eating
Narcolepsy	Linked to obesity
Night (nocturnal) eating syndrome	Eating at night with preserved consciousness
Obstructive sleep apnea	Linked to obesity
Prader-Willi syndrome	Hypersomnia; hyperphagia
Sleep-related eating disorder	Unconscious or partially conscious eating during sleep

appetite whereas ghrelin, a hormone secreted by the stomach, increases appetite. The concentration of both hormones increases during sleep. Sleep deprivation results in decreased secretion of leptin and increased secretion of ghrelin, which results in increased appetite and weight gain (Table 2). Leptin also increases in patients with obstructive sleep apnea. There are many clinical conditions in which a relation exists between sleep and eating behaviors (Table 3).

REFERENCES

1. Aserinsky E, Kleitman N. Regularly occurring periods of eye motility, and concomitant phenomena, during sleep. Science 1953; 118: 273–4.
2. Silber MH, Ancoli-Israel S, Bonnet MH, et al. The visual scoring of sleep in adults. J Clin Sleep Med 2007; 3: 121–31.
3. Ohayon MM, Carskadon MA, Guilleminault C, Vitiello MV. Meta-analysis of quantitative sleep parameters from childhood to old age in healthy individuals: developing normative sleep values across the human lifespan. Sleep 2004; 27: 1255–73.
4. Szymusiak R, McGinty D. Hypothalamic regulation of sleep and arousal. Ann N Y Acad Sci 2008; 1129: 275–86.
5. Saper CB, Scammell TE, Lu J. Hypothalamic regulation of sleep and circadian rhythms. Nature 2005; 437: 1257–63.
6. Boeve BF, Silber MH, Saper CB, et al. Pathophysiology of REM sleep behaviour disorder and relevance to neurodegenerative disease. Brain 2007; 130: 2770–88.
7. Steriade M. Brain Electrical Activity and Sensory Processing During Waking and Sleep States. In: Kryger MH, Roth T, Dement WC, editors. Principles and Practice of Sleep Medicine. 4th ed. Philadelphia (PA): Elsevier Saunders, 2005. p. 101–19.
8. Siegel JM. REM Sleep. In: Kryger MH, Roth T, Dement WC, editors. Principles and Practice of Sleep Medicine. 4th ed. Philadelphia (PA): Elsevier Saunders, 2005. p. 120–35.
9. Lu J, Sherman D, Devor M, Saper CB. A putative flip-flop switch for control of REM sleep. Nature 2006; 441:589–94.
10. Vitaterna MH, Pinto LH, Turek FW. Molecular Genetic Basis for Mammalian Circadian Rhythms. In: Kryger MH, Roth T, Dement WC, editors. Principles and Practice of Sleep Medicine. 4th ed. Philadelphia (PA): Elsevier Saunders, 2005. p. 363–74.
11. Czeisler CA, Duffy JF, Shanahan TL, et al. Stability, precision, and near-24-hour period of the human circadian pacemaker. Science 1999; 284: 2177–81.
12. Hankins MW, Peirson SN, Foster RG. Melanopsin: an exciting photopigment. Trends Neurosci 2008; 31: 27–36.
13. Szymusiak R, Gvilia I, McGinty D. Hypothalamic control of sleep. Sleep Med 2007; 8: 291–301.
14. Ekirch AR. At Day's Close: Night in Times Past. New York: Norton, 2005.
15. Rechtschaffen A, Bergmann BM, Everson CA, Kushida CA, Gilliland MA. Sleep deprivation in the rat: X. Integration and discussion of the findings. Sleep 1989; 12: 68–87.
16. Van Dongen HP, Maislin G, Mullington JM, Dinges DF. The cumulative cost of additional wakefulness: dose-response effects on neurobehavioral functions and sleep physiology from chronic sleep restriction and total sleep deprivation. Sleep 2003; 26: 117–26.

5

Diagnostic Tools in Sleep Medicine

Timothy I. Morgenthaler, MD, and Michael H. Silber, MBChB, FCP (SA)

ABBREVIATIONS

EEG, electroencephalogram

EMG, electromyogram; electromyography

ESS, Epworth Sleepiness Scale

MSLT, multiple sleep latency test

MWT, maintenance of wakefulness test

NREM, non–rapid eye movement

OSA, obstructive sleep apnea

PSG, polysomnography

REM, rapid eye movement

The field of sleep medicine has evolved slowly over the past half-century from a somewhat obscure branch of physiology to a mature medical specialty. The discovery of the electroencephalogram (EEG) for use in humans in 1929 (1) was followed shortly by the recording of brain electrical activity during sleep and by the first classification of sleep rhythms (2). After rapid eye movement (REM) sleep was discovered in 1953 (3), appreciation grew for the full spectrum of sleep-related changes in brain, eye, and muscle electrical activity. However, the application of these findings to clinical sleep disorders took another one to two decades. In the 1960s the relation of narcolepsy to premature intrusion of REM sleep (4) and sleepwalking to arousals from non–rapid eye movement (NREM) sleep was recognized (5), and the first descriptions of sleep apnea were published (6,7). The early 1970s saw the development of the first clinical sleep laboratories, which relied on polysomnography (PSG) as the main diagnostic tool. Today, to reach accurate diagnoses and plan specific treatments, comprehensive sleep medicine centers use, as appropriate, careful histories from patients and observers, quantitative scales, physical examination findings, laboratory PSG, daytime nap studies (multiple sleep latency test [MSLT] and maintenance of wakefulness test [MWT]), wrist actigraphy, and portable sleep studies.

QUANTITATIVE SCALES

Quantitative scales are vital diagnostic tools in sleep medicine. Many of these are used to assess the degree of sleepiness, including the Epworth Sleepiness Scale (ESS) (8), the Stanford Sleepiness Scale (9), and the Ullanlinna Narcolepsy Scale (10). The ESS (Figure 1) is the most widely used and has a high level of test-retest reliability. However, it correlates poorly with MSLT data, presumably measuring different facets of sleepiness.

CLINICAL PREDICTION RULES

Several clinical prediction rules have been developed to screen populations for sleep-disordered breathing and to act as decision aids in determining which persons merit further testing or monitoring. Among the more commonly used are the Berlin Questionnaire and that of Flemons et al (11,12). The Berlin Questionnaire has been validated in a general practice setting, showing a sensitivity of 87%, a specificity of 78%, a positive predictive value of 90%, and a likelihood ratio of 3.79 in predicting patients who have a measured apnea-hypopnea index of 5 or greater. It is widely used in research for case finding, and it has been found somewhat useful in screening preoperative populations to detect high risk for obstructive sleep apnea (OSA). The Flemons model takes into consideration the patient's neck circumference, history of snoring and snorting or choking during sleep, and history of hypertension. Patients who score at high risk have an 81% posttest probability of having OSA compared with 17% for those scoring at low risk (Figure 2) (13). Currently, none of the clinical prediction rules is sufficient to either exclude or diagnose OSA. However, they may be combined with clinical judgment to prioritize the need or urgency for testing.

POLYSOMNOGRAPHY

Comprehensive PSG is a technique used to assess multiple physiological parameters over the course of a night's sleep in a sleep laboratory (Table 1) (14). In modern sleep centers, the sleep rooms are designed to resemble small hotel rooms with a comfortable, bedroom-like atmosphere to avoid the typical clinical appearance of hospital rooms (Figure 3). In a standard study (Table 2), brain electrical activity is measured with 3 EEG derivations, eye movement activity with 2 electro-oculogram derivations, and muscle activity with surface electromyogram (EMG) derivations recorded from the chin and anterior tibial muscles. Other channels assess respiratory activity: surrogate measures of airflow include oronasal thermocouples and nasal pressure monitors; thoracic and abdominal inductance plethysmography measures chest and abdominal movement; pulse oximetry measures oxyhemoglobin saturation; and a microphone records the intensity of snoring. The electrocardiogram is recorded. Optional additional channels can record end-tidal or transcutaneous carbon dioxide levels, esophageal pH or pressure, body position, penile tumescence, and additional EEG activity if nocturnal seizures are suspected. Signals are appropriately filtered and displayed using digital polygraphs (Figure 4 and Figure 5).

EEG derivations record the differences between cerebral electric potentials at two sites on the head. A minimum of three

Epworth Sleepiness Scale

How likely are you to doze off or fall asleep in the following situations, in contrast to feeling just tired? This refers to your usual way of life in recent times. Even if you have not done some of these things recently, try to work out how they would have affected you. Use the following scale to choose the most appropriate number for each situation:

0 = No chance
1 = Slight chance
2 = Moderate chance
3 = High chance

Situation	Chance of Dozing
Sitting and reading	_____
Watching TV	_____
Sitting inactive in a public place (e.g., a theater or a meeting)	_____
As a passenger in a car for an hour without a break	_____
Lying down to rest in the afternoon when circumstances permit	_____
Sitting and talking to someone	_____
Sitting quietly after a lunch without alcohol	_____
In a car, while stopped for a few minutes in traffic	_____

Figure 1 Epworth Sleepiness Scale. The Epworth Sleepiness Scale is a questionnaire that measures the degree of sleepiness on a scale of 0 to 24. The upper limit of normal is generally considered to be 10 to 11 points. The Epworth Sleepiness Scale has acceptable test-retest reliability. However, its poor correlation with multiple sleep latency tests suggests that it may be measuring a different component of sleepiness. (From Johns MW [8]. [Used with permission.])

Calculation of the Modified Sleep Apnea Clinical Score

Measure:
• Neck circumference, cm

+

Add:
• 3 cm for snoring >3 nights per week
• 3 cm for witnessed apneas or choking
• 4 cm for hypertension

=

Adjusted neck circumference=
• ≤43 cm is low risk (17% pretest probability)
• 43–47.9 cm is intermediate risk
• ≥48 is high risk (81% pretest probability)

Figure 2 Clinical Prediction Rule for Obstructive Sleep Apnea: The Modified Sleep Apnea Clinical Score. To obtain the Modified Sleep Apnea Clinical Score, one begins with the neck circumference (in cm), and then adds points as indicated in the diagram if the patient snores for more than 3 nights per week, has nocturnal choking or apneic pauses to breathing, or has hypertension (treated or untreated). When the sum is <43, the risk of having obstructive sleep apnea (judged by an AHI ≥5 on polysomnography) is low (posttest probability of 17%). When the sum is ≥48, the risk is high, with a posttest probability of 81%. Such high-risk patients may be good candidates for portable home sleep studies, depending on other clinical circumstances. For comparison, clinical judgment by sleep specialists alone has an estimated specificity of 70% to 80%. (Data from Flemons WW et al [23].)

Table 1 Indications for polysomnography

Evaluation of suspected sleep–disordered breathing
    Initial diagnosis
    Titration of positive airway pressure therapy
    Follow-up of surgical or dental appliance therapy
    Follow-up after substantial changes in weight
    Evaluation of sleep symptoms in patients with neuromuscular diseases
Evaluation of excessive daytime sleepiness suspected to be due to narcolepsy or idiopathic hypersomnia
Evaluation of suspected periodic limb movement disorder
Evaluation of some suspected parasomnias
    Violent or potentially injurious behaviors
    Atypical features with diagnostic uncertainty, especially if seizures are possible
    Situations with forensic implications
Evaluation of select cases of persistent insomnia
    Suspected movement or respiratory disorder as the cause
    Failure to respond to behavioral or pharmacological treatment

Data from Kushida (14).

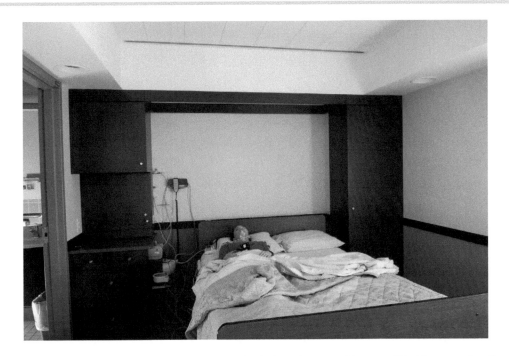

Figure 3 Sleep Recording Room. A typical sleep recording room is designed to resemble a small hotel room rather than a hospital room. Attention is paid to the comfort of the mattress and to the general ambience of the surroundings. A private bathroom is generally available, and the room has adequate soundproofing. A video camera allows a technologist to monitor the patient, who can use a bellpull to summon assistance, if necessary.

Table 2 Usual physiological parameters measured by polysomnography

System	Parameters
Neurological	Electroencephalogram
	Electro-oculogram
	Electromyogram
	Submental
	Anterior tibial
Respiratory	Airflow (both sensors required)
	Oronasal air temperature
	Nasal air pressure
	Respiratory effort
	Oxyhemoglobin saturation
	Upper airway sound
Cardiac	Electrocardiogram

derivations is used to sample potentials over the frontal, central, and occipital areas with one of two montages (a series of derivations) (Figure 6). K complexes and slow waves are maximally represented over the frontal region, sleep spindles over the central region, and waking alpha rhythm over the occipital region (see Chapter 4 on "The Physiology of Sleep"). The electro-oculogram derivations record changes in the corneoretinal potentials of the eyeball, allowing the direction and speed of eye movements to be measured (Figure 7). Slow eye movements, usually horizontal, can be observed in light (stage N1) NREM sleep, whereas rapid, irregular eye movements are characteristic of REM sleep. EMG activity falls to a minimum level during REM sleep. The EMG channels also record sleep

phenomena such as periodic limb movements and the abnormal motor activity of REM sleep behavior disorder, sleepwalking, and bruxism.

Considerable quantitative information can be obtained from an all-night PSG (Figure 8). This includes the distribution of sleep stages throughout the night, scored in 30-second intervals called *epochs*. Formal rules for scoring each stage have been developed (Table 3) (15). In addition, the frequency of arousals, respiratory events, and periodic limb movements is calculated, as well as parameters of sleep duration, timing, and continuity. Qualitative information includes the presence of parasomnias, seizure activity, cardiac arrhythmias, and intrusion of alpha frequencies into NREM sleep.

MULTIPLE SLEEP LATENCY TEST

The MSLT is a test of sleepiness (16). Patients are offered 4 or 5 nap opportunities at 2-hour intervals over the course of a day. The patient lies in bed in a dark quiet room and tries to sleep. The time from lights out until the first epoch of sleep is measured, and the mean sleep latency is calculated. If the patient does not sleep, the test is terminated after 20 minutes and an arbitrary sleep latency of 20 minutes is assigned. If the patient does fall asleep within 20 minutes, the nap opportunity continues for 15 minutes after sleep onset to assess whether REM sleep occurs (see Figure 11 in Chapter 7 on "Narcolepsy"). In between naps, the patient engages in quiet activities but is not allowed to exercise or sleep. The MSLT is usually performed the day after a night of PSG. For meaningful results, it is

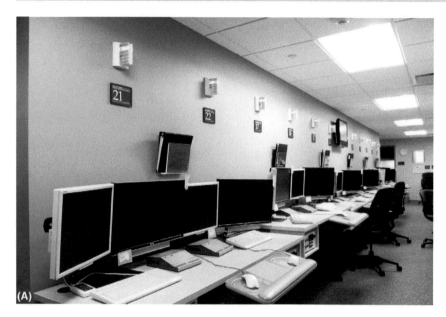

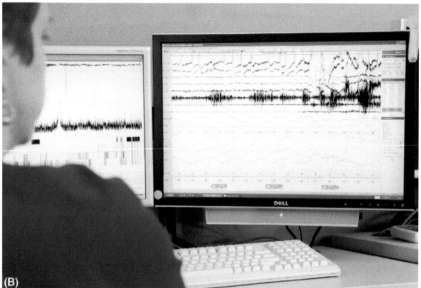

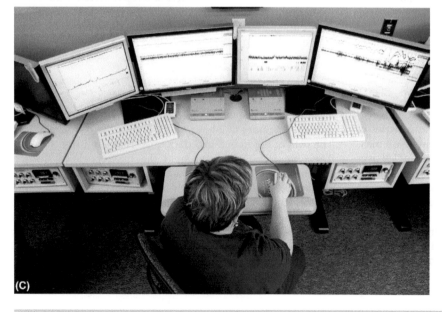

Figure 4 Sleep Laboratory Control Room. (A) All sleep studies being performed in a sleep laboratory are monitored from a control room. (B) Technologists monitor the sleep and well-being of patients in real time with the help of video cameras and microphones in the sleep recording rooms and a continuous display of physiological variables on the computer monitors. (C) Two patients can be monitored by a single technologist at one console. The technologist can communicate with the patients by microphone and can alter the settings of positive airway pressure devices without entering the sleeping rooms. However, the control room is situated in close proximity to the sleeping rooms, which allows technologists to rapidly assist the patients, if necessary.

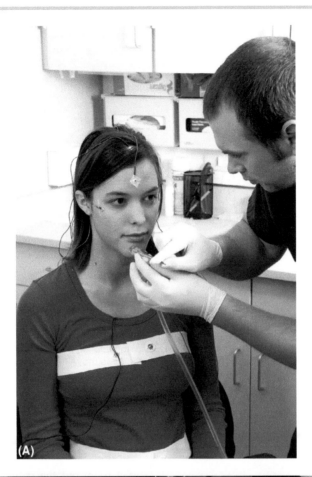

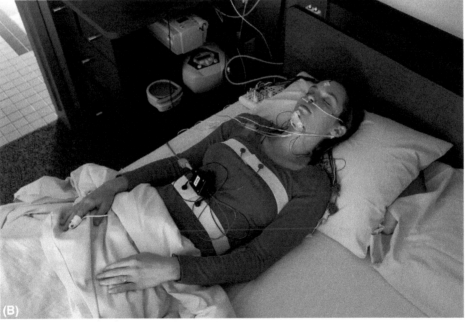

Figure 5 Sensors Used in Polysomnography. (A) Prior to the sleep study, the technologist applies sensors to monitor multiple physiological signals. The sensors include metal disk electrodes to record electroencephalographic, electro-oculographic, and electromyographic data, as well as nasal pressure monitors, chest and abdominal bands to record movements associated with breathing, electrocardiographic electrodes, a finger oximeter, and a microphone to record snoring or vocalization. (B) Despite the many wires, the patient can change position at will and can move about freely in bed. If the patient needs to get up from the bed, a technologist can be summoned to temporarily disconnect the sensors.

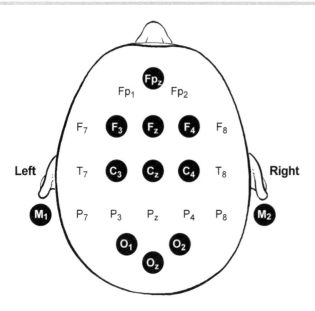

Figure 6 Electroencephalograph Derivations Used in Polysomnography. This illustration indicates the usual electroencephalography (EEG) electrodes (circled) that are used in routine polysomnography. Electrodes are placed according to the international 10-20 system. Three EEG derivations (linked pairs of electrodes) are used, monitoring the frontal (F), central (C), and occipital (O) regions. The recommended derivations are F_4-M_1, C_4-M_1, and O_2-M_1. Acceptable alternative derivations are F_z-C_z, C_z-O_z, and C_4-M_1. Fp indicates prefrontal; M, mastoid; P, parietal; T, temporal.

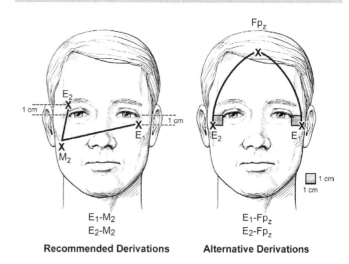

Figure 7 Electro-oculography Derivations Used in Polysomnography. This illustration indicates recommended derivations (E_1-M_2 and E_2-M_2) and acceptable alternative derivations (E_1-Fp_z and E_2-Fp_z) for recording eye movements. Eye movements are assessed by recording changes in the difference between the positive corneal potentials and the negative retinal potentials of the eyeball as the eyes move in various directions. E indicates eye; Fp, prefrontal; M, mastoid.

important to ensure that the patient has had adequate amounts of sleep for the week before the test and is not taking medications, including most psychotropic drugs, which can affect the outcome.

Normal mean sleep latency is greater than 10 minutes. Less than 5 minutes generally indicates excessive daytime sleepiness, whereas values between 5 and 10 minutes fall along a continuum, with the lower the value, the greater the probability of pathologic sleepiness (17). Most patients with narcolepsy will have a mean sleep latency of <8 minutes (18). The presence of REM sleep occurring within 15 minutes after sleep onset (sleep-onset REM) in two or more naps (16) is considered to be the neurophysiological marker of narcolepsy, but it can also be due to abrupt withdrawal from REM-suppressant medication, such as stimulants and antidepressants, moderate or severe OSA (19), or sleep deprivation (see Figure 11 in Chapter 7 on "Narcolepsy").

MAINTENANCE OF WAKEFULNESS TEST

The MWT is a variant of the MSLT used to measure the ability to remain awake (16). It is not a diagnostic test for sleepiness but rather provides objective data regarding the response to treatment of patients with disorders of hypersomnia. For example, it can play a role in determining whether patients with treated OSA can return safely to flying a plane or driving a school bus. The MWT is also conducted in a relatively dark quiet room but the patient sits up in bed with the back and head supported by a headrest. Instead of being asked to fall asleep, the patient is asked to remain awake. Each of four tests lasts 40 minutes and the mean unequivocal sleep latency (three consecutive epochs of stage N1 sleep or one epoch of any other stage) is calculated (Figure 9). Normal mean sleep latency on the MWT is 30.4 minutes, but the data are not normally distributed and 42% of all subjects remain awake for 40 minutes on all four tests (17,20). A study determining the ability of the MWT to predict simulated driving performance in patients with OSA suggested that a mean latency of 19 minutes or less correlated with driving impairment (21). Another study found that subjects with a mean latency of ≤33 minutes demonstrated increased errors driving along real roads (22). Although no consensus has been reached, current data suggest that patients with a latency of ≤19 minutes are unacceptably sleepy, whereas those with a latency in the 20- to 33-minute range may also carry a risk of driving impairment.

ACTIGRAPHY

An actigraph is a small device on a wristband worn by the patient like a wristwatch for 1 to 2 weeks (Figure 10). This device measures the number of wrist movements that occur over each 1-minute epoch. When the patient sleeps, movements reduce to a minimum and thus periods of apparent quiescence are interpreted as probable sleep (Figure 11). Conversely, periods of high activity are considered to represent wakefulness. Of course, the actigraphic appearance of lying quietly awake may mimic that of sleep, whereas active movements of

Date of Study: 9/14/09   Age: 59 years   Gender: Female

Variables Recorded: EEG, EOG, tibial and submental EMG, ECG, airflow by nasal pressure and thermocouple, chest wall motion by inductive plethysmograph, sonograph, pulse oximetry

Sleep Architecture

Start Time:	09/14/2009 22:41:46
End Time:	02/15/2009 6:40:12
	Minutes
Total Recording Time	443.5
Sleep Efficiency (TST/TRT)	82%
Initial sleep latency	7.0
Initial REM latency	65.5
Wake after sleep onset	81.0 %TST
Stage N1	30.0 8
Stage N2	163.0 45
Stage N3	79.5 22
Stage REM	91 25
Total sleep time (TST)	363.5

Disordered Breathing Profile

Frequency/Sleep Hr

Event Type Index	NREM	REM	TST
Central Apnea	0	0	0
Obstructive Apnea	0	0	0
Mixed Apnea	0	0	0
Hypopnea	5	27	11
Apnea/Hypopnea	**5**	**27**	**11**
Respiratory Effort Related Arousals	3	2	3
Respiratory Disturbance	**8**	**29**	**14**

Mean duration (seconds) of apneas/hypopneas   18

Cardiac Rhythm Abnormalities:
None

EEG Abnormalities:
None

Self Administered Medications:
None

Technical Comments:
None

CPAP Mask Size:
Not applicable

Arousal Profile

Arousal Index (#/hr)	Movement Related (%)	Breathing Related (%)
19	3	58

Effect of Body Position

	Sleep Time		AHI		RERA Index	
	Back	Off Back	Back	Off Back	Back	Off Back
NREM	47.5	225.0	19	2	3	2
REM	0.00	91.0	-	27	3	3

	Snore Rating	
	Back	Off Back
% Sleep time	30	20
Grade (0-4)	2	1

Periodic Movement Index

PLM Index	2
PLM Arousal Index	30%

Oxygen Saturation (SpO2, %) and Heart Rate (HR)

Awake Baseline: SpO2 92   HR 75

Range: NREM 90 95   REM 80 95

	>= 90	80 – 89	70 – 79	60 – 69	< 60
%TST	95	5	0	0	0

Mean SpO2	92
Max HR (TRT)	92
Max HR (TST)	90
Mean HR (TST)	72

SUMMARY: The sleep study showed normal sleep latency and normal sleep architecture. Eleven obstructive hypopneas per hour were recorded, predominantly in the supine position and during REM sleep in the lateral position of sleep. Oxyhemoglobin saturation fell to a minimum of 80%. Sleep efficiency was low at 82%. Of 19 arousals per hour, 58% were breathing related.

CLINICAL INTERPRETATION: The study shows the presence of mild, non-positional obstructive sleep apnea resulting in oxyhemoglobin desaturation and disturbance in sleep efficiency and continuity.

Figure 8 Polysomnogram Report. This figure illustrates a typical polysomnogram report. Information is available regarding sleep time, sleep efficiency, latency to sleep, different sleep stages, arousals, body position, periodic limb movements of sleep, sleep-disordered breathing, and oxyhemoglobin saturation. AHI indicates apnea-hypopnea index; CPAP, continuous positive airway pressure; ECG, electrocardiogram; EEG, electroencephalogram; EMG, electromyogram; EOG, electro-oculogram; HR, heart rate; NREM, non–rapid eye movement; PLM, periodic limb movement; REM, rapid eye movement; RERA, respiratory effort–related arousal; TRT, total recording time; TST, total sleep time.

Table 3   Criteria for sleep staging

Parameter	Sleep stage				
	W	N1	N2	N3	REM
EEG	Alpha or low amplitude, mixed frequency	Low amplitude, mixed frequency; predominantly theta	K complexes (not associated with arousals) and/or sleep spindles	$\geq$20% 0.5-2 Hz activity	Low amplitude, mixed frequency; may be sawtooth waves
EOG	Blinks and voluntary REM	Slow eye movements	None or slow eye movements	None	REM
EMG	High	Usually lower than in stage W	As in stage N1	As in stage N2, or lower	Low or absent; transient muscle activity

Abbreviations: EEG, electroencephalogram; EMG, electromyogram; EOG, electro-oculogram; REM, rapid eye movement; W, wakefulness.

Age 39 Sex M
Date of Study: 05/10/2009

Maintenance of Wakefulness Test

Nap Time	Initial Sleep Latency, min[a]	Unequivocal Sleep Latency, min[b]	Total Sleep, min
9:02	40	40	0
11:05	40	40	0
13:00	30	30.5	0.5
15:06	36	37	1.0
Mean	36.5	36.9	

[a]First epoch scored with any sleep stage.
[b]First epoch contiguous with >75 seconds of stage I or >30 seconds of any stage plus sleep spindles, K complexes, or REM (rapid eye movement) sleep.

Summary:
A maintenance of wakefulness test was performed following a night with the patient wearing CPAp set at 10 cm water pressure. The patient did not fall asleep on the first or second nap opportunities. He fell asleep at 30 minutes on the third nap opportunity and 36 minutes on the fourth nap opportunity. The mean initial sleep latency was 36.5 minutes.

Clinical Interpretation:
The ability of the patient was able to maintain alertness is within normal limits.

Figure 9 Maintenance of Wakefulness Test Report. This report illustrates typical findings in a patient undergoing a maintenance of wakefulness test to assess the effectiveness of continuous positive airway pressure therapy for sleep apnea. The mean sleep latency of 36.5 minutes is well within acceptable limits. A mean latency of <20 minutes suggests impairment in the ability to sustain wakefulness. CPAp indicates continuous positive airway pressure.

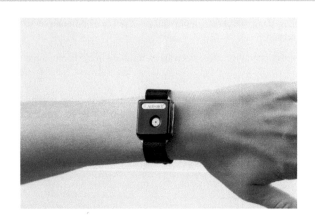

Figure 10 Actigraph. An actigraph is a small device that monitors movement. It is worn on the wrist throughout the day and night and is removed only when the patient is bathing or swimming. An actigraph is generally worn for 1 to 2 weeks. The resultant tracing provides a surrogate measure of wakefulness and sleep and is generally correlated with a sleep log kept by the patient.

the arm during sleep may mimic the appearance of wakefulness. Nevertheless, actigraphy is a valid technique for measuring total sleep time and sleep-wake patterns in normal subjects and in patients with many types of sleep disorders (23). Actigraphy is useful in characterizing the sleep patterns of patients with insomnia, including insomnia with depression, and in assisting in the diagnosis of circadian rhythm disorders, such as delayed sleep phase disorder. It is also commonly used in association with a sleep log for documenting adequate sleep time before the performance of an MSLT.

PORTABLE MONITORING

Attended complex PSG affords the opportunity for direct observations to be recorded by a trained observer (the sleep technologist), for readjustment of any sensors that might become detatched or otherwise fouled, and for direct introduction and adjustment of any therapeutic interventions such as positive airway pressure. However, a skilled attendant increases the cost of testing and intrudes upon the privacy of the patient. Testing capacity is also limited by the number of beds with PSG equipment and by the number of technologists available in sleep laboratories. In contrast, portable monitors are being advocated as more widely available, less expensive, and capable of being used in various settings, including in the home or in another health care setting. Because many portable monitors record only a limited number of signals, the American Sleep Disorders Association has proposed a portable monitoring classification scheme to categorize the largest number of permutations possible (Table 4) (24). Unattended complex PSG (type II portable monitors) differs from PSG conducted with the type I monitor (attended complex PSG) only in that it is unattended. Lacking the benefits of attended PSG and the

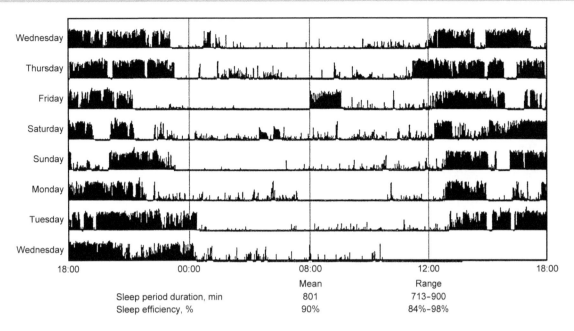

	Mean	Range
Sleep period duration, min	801	713–900
Sleep efficiency, %	90%	84%–98%

Figure 11 Display of Actigraphy Recording. This eight-day recording of rest–activity cycles shows black as activity (corresponding approximately to wakefulness) and white as rest (corresponding approximately to sleep). This patient has a variable bedtime and a long sleep period of more than 12 hours. On Friday a period of apparent wakefulness is present between 8 and 9 AM. Estimated sleep periods and sleep efficiency as calculated by the algorithm are shown.

Table 4 AASM classification of types of monitors for evaluation of sleep apnea[a]

Monitors	Signals recorded	Position	Leg movements	Interventions possible
Type I	≥ 7 Parameters, including EEG, chin EMG, ECG, airflow, respiratory effort, oximetry	Yes	Yes	Yes
Type II	≥ 7 Parameters, including EEG, chin EMG, heart rate or ECG monitor, airflow, respiratory effort, oximetry	Yes	Yes	No
Type III	≥ 4 Parameters, including ventilation or airflow (at least two channels of respiratory movement, or respiratory movement and airflow), heart rate or ECG, oximetry	Yes	Maybe	No
Type IV	1-2 Parameters, typically oximetry plus heart rate or airflow	Yes	Yes	Yes

Abbreviations: AASM, American Academy of Sleep Medicine; ECG, electrocardiogram; EEG, electroencephalogram; EMG, electromyogram.
[a]With a minimum of six hours of recording.

convenient and less complicated hookups of type III and type IV monitors, type II devices are most often used in research settings.

The most commonly used portable monitors are type III (Figure 12) and type IV. Such a device may be configured to provide continuous data from oximetry, airflow (using either thermocouple or nasal pressure), respiratory impedence plethysmography, snoring, body position, and actigraphy (Figure 13). The most common type IV monitor is ambulatory pulse oximetry, which provides a continuous recording of oxygen saturation (Figure 14). Pulse oximetry is not recommended as a diagnostic test for OSA, but it may be used to screen for sleep-disordered breathing in patients at high risk (such as those with heart failure), and to assess the impact on oxygenation of therapeutic interventions such as continuous positive airway pressure.

Type III portable monitors may be used as part of the evaluation strategy for patients with a high pretest probability of having moderate or severe OSA (see Chapter 6 on "Sleep-Related Breathing Disorders"). Their validity in patients with comorbid conditions such as central sleep apnea, obstructive lung disease, hypoventilation disorders, or neuromuscular disease has not been firmly established. Otherwise, they are suitable for diagnostic studies that do not require intervention and for reassessing the efficacy of therapy in patients previously diagnosed with sleep apnea and treated for it. Studies conducted with portable monitors experience rates of lead failure or data loss as high as 16%. Nonetheless, OSA may be diagnosed with confidence when the clinical picture suggests a high probability of OSA and an acceptable type III portable monitor study reveals more than five apneas and hypopneas per hour of recording (24).

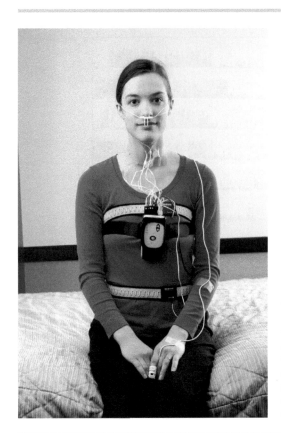

Figure 12 Type III Portable Monitor. This type III portable respiratory monitor (Embletta; Embla, Broomfield, Colorado) is configured to record airflow using a nasal pressure transducer (via the nasal cannula) and a thermocouple (located over the nares and mouth), respiratory chest and abdominal excursion with respiratory impedance plethysmography, and oximetry with a finger probe. The recording device, strapped to the chest, also serves as a position monitor (able to indicate supine, left, right, prone, and upright positions) and an actigraph. This and other marketed devices may also have additional sensors, such as leg motion sensors. The device may be self-applied, and it can be used in various settings.

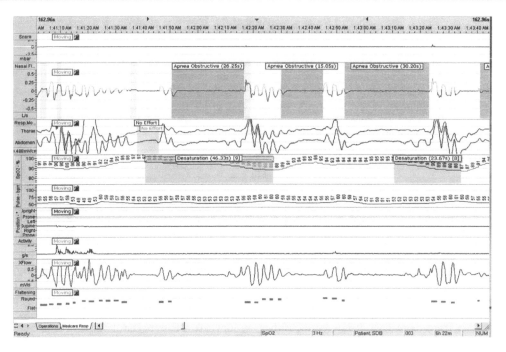

Figure 13 Type III Portable Monitor Recording. This recording was obtained using an Embletta respiratory monitor (Embla, Broomfield, Colorado) worn by a patient suspected of having obstructive sleep apnea. From top to bottom, tracings are: 1) snoring (may be derived from a microphone or from high-frequency oscillations of a nasal pressure transducer; here, not showing snoring that was actually present); 2) nasal pressure as an indicator of flow; 3) thoracic and abdominal excursion with impedance plethysmography; 4) finger pulse oximetry; 5) pulse rate from pulse oximetry; 6) position derived from a gravitometric sensor located in the recording box (see Figure 12); 7) movement from the actigraph located in the recording box (see Figure 12); 8) XFlow, a summation of the thoracic and abdominal plethysmographic recordings; and 9) the flattening index, an indicator of upper airway obstruction, with "flat" indicating more obstruction than "round." The pink markings denote apneas detected in the flow channel that are considered obstructive because of the ongoing (and at times paradoxical) effort shown in the thorax and abdominal channels. Desaturations (in gray) are marked by algorithm or manually. Excessive movement, suggesting wakefulness or arousal, is marked in the first moments of this tracing. The "roundest" (least obstructed) flow is observed during the recovery breaths following obstructive apneas.

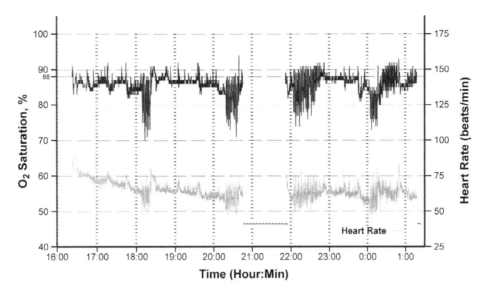

Figure 14 Ambulatory Overnight Oximetry. This oximetry tracing is from a patient suspected of having obstructive sleep apnea because of symptoms of snoring and obesity, but who reported no other symptoms of sleep apnea. The recording was requested to help prioritize the decision of whether to pursue more definitive testing in view of other health care concerns being addressed at the time of the evaluation (preoperative assessment for total knee arthroplasty in a patient with interstitial lung disease; awake upright arterial oxygen saturation, 90.5%). The tracing shows an abnormal supine baseline oxygen saturation averaging 87% with repetitive oscillatory desaturations (desaturations of at least 4% from baseline, shown in red, totaled 179 over 7 hours and 48 minutes of valid recording time, for an oxygen desaturation index of 22.9 per hour). Some of the deeper desaturations clump together and occur about every two hours, suggesting a worsening of sleep-disordered breathing with the transition to rapid eye movement sleep or with a change in position. The pulse rate is highly variable during these deeper desaturations as one might find with rapid eye movement or with the tachycardia-bradycardia phenomenon seen with obstructive apneas. The recording period (starting at 16:25 hours and ending at 01:20 hours) seems advanced for sleep consistent with the shift work of the patient. Like many ambulatory portable monitor recordings, this one has data loss (scalloped line [∼ ∼ ∼]) between 20:45 and 21:45 hours). Surgery plans for the patient were delayed while other aspects of his pulmonary and sleep health were evaluated.

REFERENCES

1. Berger H. Uber das elektrenkephalogramm des menschen. Arch Psychiatr 1929; 87: 527–70.
2. Loomis AL, Harvey EN, Hobart GA. Cerebral states during sleep, as studied by human brain potentials. J Exp Psychol 1937; 21: 127–44.
3. Aserinsky E, Kleitman N. Regularly occurring periods of eye motility, and concomitant phenomena, during sleep. Science 1953; 118: 273–4.
4. Vogel G. Studies in psychophysiology of dreams. III. The dream of narcolepsy. Arch Gen Psychiatry 1960; 3: 421–8.
5. Broughton RJ. Sleep disorders: disorders of arousal? Enuresis, somnambulism, and nightmares occur in confusional states of arousal, not in "dreaming sleep". Science 1968; 159: 1070–8.
6. Gastaut H, Tassinari CA, Duron B. Etude polygraphique des manifestations épisodiques (hypniques et respiratoires), diurnes et nocturnes, du syndrome de Pickwick. Rev Neurol 1965; 112: 568–79.
7. Jung R, Kuhlo W. Neurophysiological studies of abnormal night sleep and the Pickwickian syndrome. Prog Brain Res 1965; 18: 140–59.
8. Johns MW. A new method for measuring daytime sleepiness: the Epworth Sleepiness Scale. Sleep 1991; 14: 540–5.
9. Hoddes E, Zarcone V, Smythe H, Phillips R, Dement WC. Quantification of sleepiness: a new approach. Psychophysiology 1973; 10: 431–6.
10. Hublin C, Kaprio J, Partinen M, Koskenvuo M, Heikkila K. The Ullanlinna Narcolepsy Scale: validation of a measure of symptoms in the narcoleptic syndrome. J Sleep Res 1994; 3: 52–9.

11. Flemons WW. Clinical practice: obstructive sleep apnea. N Engl J Med 2002; 347: 498–504.
12. Netzer NC, Stoohs RA, Netzer CM, Clark K, Strohl KP. Using the Berlin Questionnaire to identify patients at risk for the sleep apnea syndrome. Ann Intern Med 1999; 131: 485–91.
13. Flemons WW, Whitelaw WA, Brant R, Remmers JE. Likelihood ratios for a sleep apnea clinical prediction rule. Am J Respir Crit Care Med 1994; 150(5 Pt 1):1279–85.
14. Kushida CA, Littner MR, Morgenthaler T, et al. Practice parameters for the indications for polysomnography and related procedures: an update for 2005. Sleep 2005; 28: 499–521.
15. Iber C, Ancoli-Israel S, Chessonn A, Quan SF for the American Academy of Sleep Medicine. The AASM Manual for the Scoring of Sleep and Associated Events: Rules, Terminology and Technical Specifications. Westchester (IL): American Academy of Sleep Medicine, 2007.
16. Littner MR, Kushida C, Wise M, et al; Standards of Practice Committee of the American Academy of Sleep Medicine. Practice parameters for clinical use of the multiple sleep latency test and the maintenance of wakefulness test. Sleep 2005; 28: 113–21.
17. Arand D, Bonnet M, Hurwitz T, Mitler M, Rosa R, Sangal RB. The clinical use of the MSLT and MWT. Sleep 2005; 28: 123–44.
18. American Academy of Sleep Medicine. The International Classification of Sleep Disorders: Diagnostic and Coding Manual. 2nd ed. Westchester (IL): American Academy of Sleep Medicine, 2005.
19. Aldrich MS, Chervin RD, Malow BA. Value of the multiple sleep latency test (MSLT) for the diagnosis of narcolepsy. Sleep 1997; 20: 620–9.

20. Doghramji K, Mitler MM, Sangal RB, et al. A normative study of the maintenance of wakefulness test (MWT). Electroencephalogr Clin Neurophysiol 1997; 103: 554–62.

21. Sagaspe P, Taillard J, Chaumet G, et al. Maintenance of wakefulness test as a predictor of driving performance in patients with untreated obstructive sleep apnea. Sleep 2007; 30: 327–30.

22. Philip P, Sagaspe P, Taillard J, et al. Maintenance of wakefulness test, obstructive sleep apnea syndrome, and driving risk. Ann Neurol 2008; 64: 410–6.

23. Morgenthaler T, Alessi C, Friedman L, et al; Standards of Practice Committee; American Academy of Sleep Medicine. Practice parameters for the use of actigraphy in the assessment of sleep and sleep disorders: an update for 2007. Sleep 2007; 30: 519–29.

24. Collop NA, Anderson WM, Boehlecke B, et al; Portable Monitoring Task Force of the American Academy of Sleep Medicine. Clinical guidelines for the use of unattended portable monitors in the diagnosis of obstructive sleep apnea in adult patients. J Clin Sleep Med 2007; 3: 737–47.

6

Sleep-Related Breathing Disorders

Timothy I. Morgenthaler, MD

ABBREVIATIONS

AHI, apnea-hypopnea index

BMI, body mass index (weight in kg/height in m^2)

CPAP, continuous positive airway pressure

CSBP, Cheyne-Stokes breathing pattern

ICSD-2, *International Classification of Sleep Disorders*, 2nd edition

MAD, mandibular advancement device

NREM, non–rapid eye movement

OSAS, obstructive sleep apnea syndrome

PAP, positive airway pressure

REM, rapid eye movement

VENTILATORY CONTROL

The respiratory system is complex and responds to diverse challenges. It not only maintains homeostatic levels of Pa_{O_2}, Pa_{CO_2}, and pH over a wide range of activity levels but it also does this in spite of less continuous challenges such as speaking, breath holding, micturition, defecation, emesis, coughing, parturition, blowing out birthday candles, and singing. Control of the upper airway allows persons not only to breathe but also to phonate and eat, while either stationary or moving and while in various positions. The upper airway in humans, rather than being a bony tube of fixed diameter, is a flexible structure held patent by a balance of muscle tone and tensions. Sleep changes the respiratory control and muscle tone in the upper airway. Given the variety of challenges that the ventilatory control system must meet, it is perhaps not surprising that the system is not always successful. When abnormal breathing patterns occur during sleep, the condition is called sleep-disordered breathing. Table 1 summarizes the most common types of sleep-disordered breathing. These disorders have unique pathophysiology and typical clinical presentations, and most can be addressed with management strategies that are highly effective.

At its simplest level, the signal to breathe originates with a special set of neurons called the Bötzinger complex, which is located in the medulla (Figure 1). When unmodulated by other influences, the breathing pattern would be steady, periodic, and almost mechanical, similar to the pattern observed in patients who are entirely ventilator dependent. However, the rhythmic output of this complex is modified by the integration of inputs by at least six other neurons located primarily in the medulla, which altogether are called the respiratory control center. These neurons receive input from the Bötzinger complex and a wide variety of influences (Table 2). Many of these influences are automatic and consist of feedback from chemoreceptors and mechanoreceptors. Other inputs descend from cortical areas and attend to our desire to perform intermittent activities such as speaking or breath holding. One very important additional influence is known as the wakefulness input.

Before examining the wakefulness input, it is important to understand the automatic parts of the respiratory control system. The output of this system travels via phrenic motoneurons, spinal nerves, and cranial nerves to produce the coordinated movements of ventilation. These movements produce gas exchange that influences chemoreceptors, which in turn provide input back to the respiratory control system. In addition, the actual movements, pressure changes, and vascular dynamics of ventilation elicit responses from various mechanoreceptors and nocioceptors that are also relayed to the respiratory control system. Thus, the whole system is a classic feedback system (Figure 2). The respiratory control system is one component (i.e., the controller), and the moving parts (i.e., the muscles, lungs, chest wall, circulation, and corporeal metabolism) may be thought of as the plant. Output from the controller influences the plant and vice versa, whereas input from the plant influences the controller and vice versa.

Conceptualizing the respiratory control system this way is useful when one ponders the stability of the system. In a totally homeostatic system, there is complete balance between input and output, and the system behaves in a predictable fashion, producing rhythmic breathing, even gas exchange, and uniform neural output. However, this does not sound like real life. In real life, we must be able to respond to various perturbations or disturbances in the system. For example, what if there is a momentary increase in production of CO_2, such as may happen with exertion or a fever? What if one ascends to a high altitude, with a resulting change in the inspired fraction of oxygen? What if mucus production in the airways produces segmental atelectasis and changes ventilation/perfusion matching? Feedback systems may respond to such disturbances in one of three ways. If they do not respond at all, due to inflexibility on the part of the controller or the plant, then homeostasis will be lost entirely, with migration of the system's set-point in a constant direction away from its originally healthy one. In the case of ventilation, this could be fatal because P_{CO_2}, P_{O_2}, and pH must be regulated within a relatively small tolerance. Alternatively, the system could adjust to the disturbance to find a new safe set-point close to the healthy one by adjusting output to meet the new demand, thus dampening the result of the disturbance. Nonetheless, the system could destabilize, producing a fluctuating circumstance without finding a new stable homeostatic set-point (Figure 3).

The likelihood of the feedback system responding to a disturbance by finding a new homeostasis has been estimated

Table 1   Sleep-disordered breathing syndromes

Syndrome	Characteristics
Obstructive sleep apnea syndrome	Recurrent episodes of partial or complete upper airway obstruction during sleep. Breathing events include obstructive apneas, obstructive hypopneas, mixed apneas, and respiratory effort–related arousals.
Idiopathic central sleep apnea	Recurrent apneic episodes during sleep in the absence of upper airway obstruction or hypercapnia (hypercapnic patients are considered to have alveolar hypoventilation syndrome).
Central sleep apnea due to Cheyne-Stokes breathing pattern	Cyclic fluctuation in ventilatory pattern during sleep with periods of central apnea or hypopnea alternating with hyperpnea in a crescendo-decrescendo manner. The period of the cycles typically exceeds 45 seconds.
Central sleep apnea due to high altitude periodic breathing	Recurrent central sleep apneas primarily during NREM sleep at a frequency of more than 5 per hour occurring after ascent to 4,000 meters. Often a periodic crescendo-decrescendo pattern is noted in a period of 12 to 34 seconds.
Central sleep apnea due to a medical condition other than Cheyne-Stokes breathing pattern	Central sleep apnea in the presence of a medical condition other than heart failure believed to be its cause. Stroke, trauma, or demyelinating diseases may be the cause. In stroke, the period is typically <30 seconds. In other cases, aperiodicity may be more common.
Central sleep apnea due to drug use or substance abuse	Repetitive central apneas or periodic breathing in a patient chronically using substances, usually opioids, associated with this pattern. The pattern is often less rhythmic "ataxic breathing."
Complex sleep apnea syndrome	Patients demonstrate a predominant obstructive pattern, but when obstruction is relieved, a persistent central sleep apnea pattern is revealed.
Central sleep apnea of infancy	Patients demonstrate prolonged sleep-disordered breathing events associated with physiological compromise such as hypoxemia, bradycardia, or the need for interventions to sustain breathing.
Alveolar hypoventilation syndrome (sleep hypoventilation syndrome)	Hypercapnia and hypoxemia during sleep due to inappropriate central hypoventilation and not due exclusively to obstructive apneas and hypopneas. Diurnal hypercapnia is often present.

Abbreviation: NREM, non–rapid eye movement.

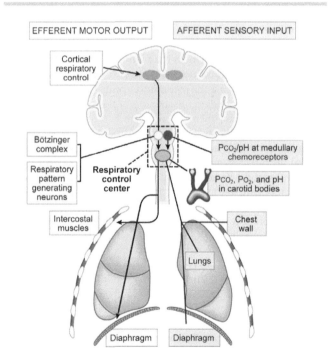

Figure 1   The Respiratory Control System. Control of ventilation is achieved by a feedback control system, with the main controlling neurons located in the medulla. The inputs to the respiratory pattern generating neurons (at right) include the rhythmic input from the Bötzinger complex and modulation from the medullary chemoreceptors, the carotid bodies, the mechanoreceptors located throughout the airway and chest wall, and the cortex. The medullary control center integrates these inputs to produce the efferent signals (at left) that control the respiratory muscles of the oropharynx, the intercostal muscles, and the diaphragm.

by determining the system's "loop gain," which is the ratio of the response to a disturbance to the magnitude of the disturbance (Figure 2). When loop gain is >1, the system is predictably prone to instability. With a loop gain of <1, the system tends to absorb disturbances more easily (Figure 3). When the components of the respiratory system are examined this way, one might be able to predict factors that would tend to destabilize the breathing pattern. For example, factors that increase the output of the ventilatory control center in response to a rise in $Paco_2$ (the hypercapnic ventilatory response) or a decline in Pao_2 (the hypoxic ventilatory response) would tend to destabilize the system. We will return to this concept during the discussion of central sleep apnea syndromes because factors that increase loop gain favor the development of many types of central sleep apnea syndrome.

Thus, at its most basic, the ventilatory control system is a classic feedback system that is further modulated by voluntary inputs from cortical regions and also strongly influenced by sleep state. During NREM (non–rapid eye movement) sleep, the ventilatory system is predominantly governed by the feedback system described above and, if undisturbed by arousal or other perturbation, it is generally rhythmic and regular. During healthy steady state breathing while asleep, blood oxygen saturation is 1% to 2% lower, and both hypercapnic responsiveness and hypoxic ventilatory responsiveness are diminished compared with those of the wake state (Figure 4). This difference in ventilatory drive between sleep and wake has been called the wakefulness input. Wakefulness input changes not only the ventilatory response curves but also the apneic threshold, that is, the $Paco_2$ below which ventilatory drive essentially ceases, thus causing centrally mediated apnea (Figure 4). Another important physiological change during sleep that may affect ventilation is the regulation of muscle tone, which is reduced in NREM sleep compared with wake and which is minimal during REM (rapid eye movement) sleep. This

Table 2 Components influencing respiratory control

I. Automatic respiratory control system
  A. Medullary respiratory center
    1. Afferents to the medullary respiratory center
      a) Chemoreceptors
        (1) Medullary chemoreceptors
          (a) Influenced predominantly by Pa_{CO_2} via changes in cerebrospinal fluid pH; to a lesser extent, influenced by Pa_{O_2}, oxygen consumption
        (2) Peripheral chemoreceptors (carotid bodies, aortic bodies)
          (a) Influenced predominantly by Pa_{O_2}
      b) Mechanoreceptors
        (1) Mechanoreceptors in the upper respiratory tract
          (a) Influenced by temperature, pressure, contact/touch, humidity, and various chemical substances
        (2) Mechanoreceptors in lower respiratory tract and lungs
          (a) Irritant receptors
            i) Respond to mechanical as well as nonspecific chemical irritation
          (b) Stretch receptors
            i) Responsible for the Hering-Breuer reflex
          (c) J receptors
            i) Stimulate ventilation in response to a variety of stimuli, including microembolization of the pulmonary circulation, pulmonary edema
        (3) Mechanoreceptors in the muscle spindles and tendon organs in the respiratory muscles
          (a) Monitor the effectiveness of the peripheral effector system
    2. Efferents from the medullary respiratory center to respiratory organs
      a) Phrenic nerve
        (1) Innervate the diaphragm
      b) Spinal nerves to the intercostal and abdominal muscles
        (1) Innervate the intercostal and abdominal muscles
      c) Cranial and spinal nerves to the upper airway
        (1) Innervate numerous muscles of the pharynx, hypopharynx, larynx, and tongue, including the genioglossals, tensor palatini, medial pterygoids, cricothyroid, and posterior cricoarytenoids
        (2) Voluntary respiratory control system
  B. Cortical neurons
    1. Voluntarily direct variability in respiratory processes, such as breath holding, coughing, or singing, while awake

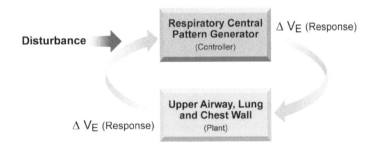

$$\text{Loop Gain} = \frac{\text{(Response to disturbance = Controller response + Plant response)}}{\text{(The disturbance itself)}}$$

Figure 2 Ventilatory Feedback Loop. The respiratory central pattern generator is the "controller" that sends signals to initiate and modulate ventilation. The primary purpose of this center is to support the physiology of the rest of the body, which altogether may be thought of as a sort of "plant" that generates useful work (e.g., labor, thought, or metabolism). The feedback from the plant influences the output of the controller, completing a classic feedback loop. Any new disturbance to the function of the plant, such as exercise, fever, a new meal, stress, upper airway obstruction, or, importantly, changes in sleep state (e.g., falling asleep or an arousal from sleep) will result in feedback from the plant. The output of the controller will, in turn, be modulated by that feedback. How much response is generated by the controller because of the disturbance is determined by the "controller gain." For example, some people may have a more marked ventilatory response to a certain degree of hypercapnia. The output of the plant in response to its input from the control center is described by the "plant gain." For example, the plant response of a patient with neuromuscular disease to a given level of output from the medullary control center may be substantially lower than that of an athletic mountain climber (see Figure 3). ΔV_E indicates change in minute ventilation.

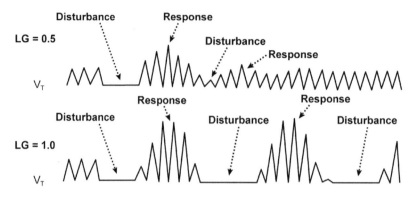

$$\text{Loop Gain} = \frac{\text{(Response to disturbance)}}{\text{(The disturbance itself)}}$$

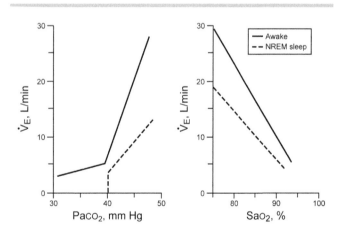

Figure 3 Loop Gain. The ratio of the response to a disturbance to the disturbance itself may be conceptualized as the loop gain (LG), a way to characterize the function of the entire feedback system (see Figure 2). In general, systems with loop gains of ≥ 1 tend toward instability, whereas those with loop gains of slightly <1 are more stable. A system with a loop gain of 0 would be an unchanging system, unable to respond to even routine challenges to homeostasis, such as walking across the room, coughing, or talking. In this hypothetical example, the disturbance is an apnea (cause unimportant). After the response thresholds are crossed, the response to the ensuing hypercapnia and hypoxemia is to increase ventilation. In the top example, with a loop gain of 0.5, the response is just enough to restore the system close to homeostasis, and steady state is achieved with only one more iteration. In the bottom example with a loop gain of 1.0, the response to the apnea overshoots homeostasis and becomes a disturbance in its own right, leading to yet another apnea and so on. Even greater swings away from equilibrium would result as the loop gain is increased to >1. V_T indicates tidal volume. (From White DP. Pathogenesis of obstructive and central sleep apnea. Am J Respir Crit Care Med 2005; 172:1363-70. [Used with permission.])

Figure 4 Ventilatory Response Curves at Steady State, Awake, and Asleep. The ventilation at a given $Paco_2$ while breathing a constant high inspiratory pressure of oxygen, is depicted at left. Below the threshold value of $Paco_2$ ≤ 40 mm H_2O, the ventilation changes only slightly with $Paco_2$ and is low during wakefulness and absent during non–rapid eye movement (NREM) sleep. This point is called the apneic threshold, and it varies a bit between wakefulness and sleep. Note that above the apneic threshold, the change in ventilation per unit change in $Paco_2$, a measure of the ventilatory drive, is lower in NREM sleep than in wakefulness. At right is depicted the eucapneic ventilatory drive related to arterial oxygen saturation (Sao_2). Note that the hypoxic ventilatory drive is also lower in NREM sleep than in wakefulness. $\dot{V}_E$ indicates minute ventilation.

reduction in muscle tone, combined with changes in ventilatory drive, helps explain the changes in minute ventilation, tidal volume, and respiratory rate that are noted across the range of sleep stages.

SLEEP-RELATED RESPIRATORY EVENTS
Obstructive Apneas and Hypopneas

Understanding ventilatory control is essential to a proper understanding of sleep-disordered breathing. However, the controller is only part of the system; the plant is also an essential component. The output of the controller instructs the ventilatory muscles to activate. However, activation must occur in a precise manner. When either the controller or the plant fails to function in a coordinated fashion, a ventilatory event results (Table 3). For example, in a situation where activation of phrenic nerves would produce an inspiratory maneuver by the diaphragms, if the output to the upper airway muscles was inadequate or ill timed, the airway would not be patent. The diaphragms would produce a negative intrathoracic pressure sufficient to promote airflow from the atmosphere into the lungs, but the closed airway would prevent that flow. This lack of airflow is called an apnea (Greek for "no breath"), and it is precisely the mechanism underlying an obstructive apnea (obstructive because it is airway obstruction that produces the apnea rather than the lack of forces sufficient to produce negative intrathoracic pressure). By convention, apneas are not counted until the absence of ventilation has lasted for at least 10 seconds (Figure 5). In the event that the airway is not totally collapsed but remains too narrow to allow normal airflow, the

Table 3 Sleep-related breathing events and their definitions

Event	Definition
Obstructive apnea	A cessation of airflow for at least 10 seconds, during which there is effort to breathe.
Central apnea	A cessation of airflow for at least 10 seconds, during which there is no effort to breathe.
Mixed apnea	A cessation of airflow for at least 10 seconds, with the event commencing as a central apnea but terminating as an obstructive apnea.
Hypopnea	An abnormal respiratory event lasting at least 10 seconds, with at least a 30% reduction in thoracoabdominal movement or airflow as compared to baseline, and with at least a 4% oxyhemoglobin desaturation. A hypopnea can be proven obstructive only with an esophageal balloon that shows increasing effort with reduced airflow, but it can often be inferred from the shape of the airflow signal or when snoring intensity increases during the event.
Respiratory effort–related arousal	A sequence of breaths with increasing respiratory effort leading to arousal from sleep. This is best demonstrated by progressively more negative esophageal pressure efforts for at least 10 seconds preceding an arousal with resumption of more normal pressures, but it often can be inferred from other measured signals.

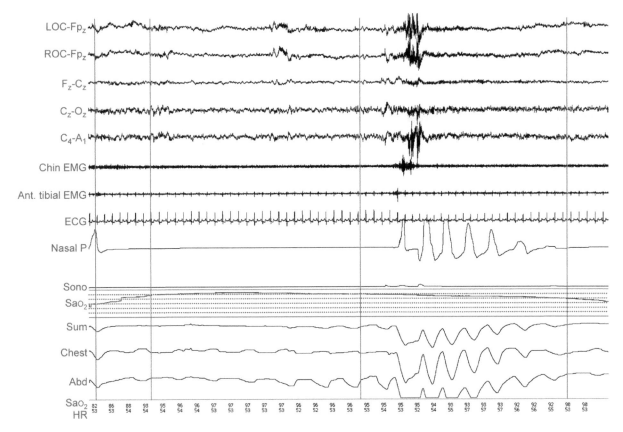

Figure 5 Obstructive Apnea. In this 60-second polysomnographic epoch of stage N2 sleep, an apnea begins almost immediately upon entering the epoch (nasal pressure tracing shows no evidence of air movement). The apnea is confirmed by the sum (Sum) of the chest and abdominal (Abd) respiratory impedance bands, which also shows no significant tidal volume during the apnea. There is clear evidence of thoracoabdominal paradox, with the Abd and chest bands moving in opposite rather than synchronous directions. The rhythm is sinus and does not demonstrate the clinically significant tachy-bradycardia often observed with more profound desaturations and longer apneas. This apnea lasts about 40 seconds. Note the abrupt resumption of ventilation (not a gradually increasing or crescendo pattern) that is characteristic of the termination of obstructive events. The arousal is practically concurrent with termination of the apnea. Unfortunately for this patient, another apnea ensues with the return to sleep. Vertical lines are 15 seconds apart; the total epoch time is 30 seconds. Abd indicates abdominal; Ant. tibial, anterior tibial muscles; ECG, electrocardiogram; EMG, electromyogram; HR, heart rate; LOC, left outer canthus; Nasal P, nasal pressure; ROC, right outer canthus; Sao$_2$, arterial oxygen saturation; Sono, sonographic microphone to record snoring; Sum, sum of the chest and abdominal respiratory impedance bands.

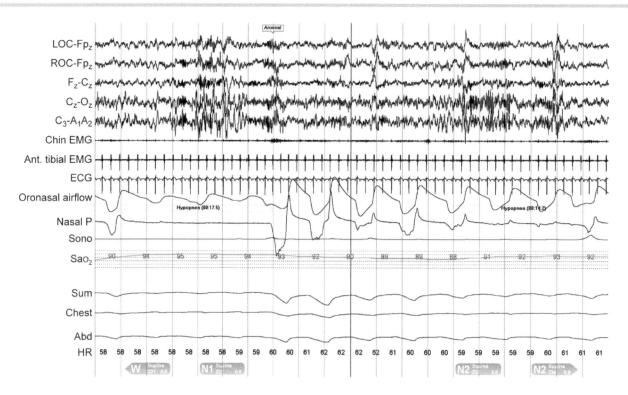

Figure 6 Hypopnea. During this 60-second epoch, a hypopnea begins at about 3 seconds into the tracing and lasts about 12 seconds. The nasal pressure transducer signal is often the most sensitive in picking up hypopneas and flow limitations. In this polysomnographic tracing, it is flat throughout the hypopnea. The thermocouple (Oronasal airflow) shows ongoing evidence of air movement, but it is of lower magnitude than surrounding breaths and is shown to be sufficient to cause a significant decline in arterial oxygen saturation (Sao_2) from 95% to 88%. Note the delay in oxygen saturation decline of about 12 seconds, which is typical of patients without clinically significant heart disease. The time between cessation of breathing and the nadir of oxygen saturation, which is called the *lung-to-finger circulation time*, is about 15 seconds in patients without heart failure in contrast to 22 to 35 seconds for patients with impaired left ventricular function (1,2). Note also the abrupt resumption of airflow at hypopnea termination, which, along with the flattening of the inspiratory breaths observed after the hypopnea, is characteristic of an obstruction. One might expect more activity in the sonographic microphone channel (Sono), but the gain may be low. To be certain of whether the hypopnea was due to upper airway obstruction or centrally mediated causes would require the use of an esophageal manometer. For explanation of labels, see Figure 5. (For more information, see Silber MH, Krahn LE, Morgenthaler TI. Sleep Medicine in Clinical Practice. New York [NY]: Taylor & Francis, 2004. p. 131-2.)

resulting inadequate tidal volumes and decline in minute ventilation define an obstructive hypopnea. A decline in ventilation could also result from reduced ventilatory control output or weak output from the ventilatory muscles. Because of this, hypopneas that are scored during clinical polysomnography without using some measure of intrathoracic pressure such as an esophageal pressure manometer are not usually classified as either obstructive or central in origin (Figure 6). Although the concept of a hypopnea is clear, the definition conventions by which events should be counted as such are more variable. Most commonly, hypopneas are defined as respiratory events with evidence of ongoing ventilatory efforts but with at least 30% reduced airflow lasting 10 seconds and sufficient enough to result in a decline in blood oxygen saturation of at least 4% (3). Apneas and hypopneas have in common three characteristics: 1) alteration in the normal ventilatory pattern that involves a reduction in airflow; 2) transience, but with each lasting at least 10 seconds; and 3) frequently, decreased oxygenation. After these events occur, ventilation resumes. The curious reader might wonder about two things. First, what signals cause ventilation to resume; and second, what happens

when it does resume? How does the ventilatory control center compensate for this disruption?

Recovering From an Obstructive Apnea or Hypopnea
Traditionally, it has been taught that an arousal from sleep is required to increase airway tone in order to open the upper airway and allow a resumption of ventilation after an obstructive apnea. However, this is not always the case. Recent studies analyzing the relationship between airway opening and arousal show a more complicated arrangement (4). The airway may be opened in response to an increase in control center output despite the absence of arousal, or it may occur at the time of arousal or even afterward (Figure 7). The signal to open the closed airway arises from the central controller, whose output may be modulated by inputs from mechanoreceptors in the lungs and airway that indicate the discrepancy between output and effect, as well as inputs from chemoreceptors indicating hypoxia or hypercapnia. Why some apneas and hypopneas are terminated by arousal, whereas others are overcome without arousal, is not entirely understood.

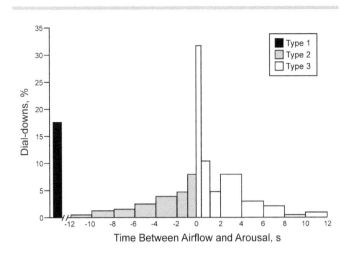

Figure 7 Time Between Onset of Airflow After an Obstructive Apnea and an Arousal. The idea that arousal is necessary to "rescue" the patient from upper airway obstruction is a logical but erroneous conclusion. Recent studies show an inconsistent relationship between the timing of arousal and upper airway opening. This graph depicts results from a study in which obstructive apneas and hypopneas were induced by the dial-down of continuous positive airway pressure in patients with obstructive sleep apnea. The time was measured from the beginning of the obstructive event until arousal and until airway opening with resumption of airflow. The graph depicts the time difference between airflow resumption and an electroencephalogram (EEG) arousal on the ordinate, and the frequency at which those time differences are observed is depicted along the abscissa. The response to induced obstructive apneas or hypopneas was assigned to one of three types on the basis of the relationship to any EEG arousal. Type 1 responses were those wherein the subjects resumed airflow without apparent arousal; type 2 responses were those involving resumption of airflow before arousal; and type 3 responses showed airflow only after arousal. Clearly, many obstructive events are terminated without arousal or before arousal (5). (From Younes [4]. [Used with permission.])

Snoring and Respiratory Effort–Related Arousals

Upper airway resistance is not constant during wake or sleep. However, as long as ventilatory effort increases or decreases in proportion to the change in resistance, airflow will remain stable. The degree of inspiratory effort can be described by the magnitude of intrathoracic pressure (as estimated by intraesophageal pressure manometry). During normal ventilation, the intrathoracic pressure required to maintain ventilation typically ranges from -5 to -35 cm H_2O, depending on the airflow needed and the upper airway resistance. The audible vibrations of the upper airway set in motion by the turbulent flow through the narrowed airway produce snoring, which can range in volume from insignificant to highly disruptive for persons sharing space with the snoring sleeper. Snoring occurs in 30% to 50% of adults older than age 50 years, and it is loud enough to be heard in an adjacent room in 5% to 10% of these adults (6). In a recent study of patients referred for sleep evaluations, snoring produced sound intensity levels that averaged 46.2 decibels and that exceeded regulatory outdoor noise limits in 12.3% of patients. Snoring is more common in patients with nasal congestion measured objectively by rhinometry (7).

Because snoring results from muscle tone–related reductions in airway dimensions, it is frequently also present in patients with apneas and hypopneas.

At times, the resistance increases so much that the ventilatory effort needed to maintain flow is great enough to stimulate an arousal from sleep. Figure 8 illustrates how a patient's increasing effort to maintain airflow results in arousing him from sleep. When the increased effort lasts 10 seconds and terminates in an arousal, the event is called a respiratory effort–related arousal.

Central Apneas

When there is no signal sent from the central respiratory controller, there is no airflow. This event, called a central apnea, is most frequent during lighter stages of sleep, particularly with the transition from wake to sleep (Figure 9). Isolated sleep-onset central apneas are not infrequent in normal sleepers because the central controller may interpret the normal $PaCO_2$ of wakefulness as too low when measured against the higher CO_2 apnea threshold of sleep. The change from wake to sleep serves as the "disturbance" to the respiratory system. As the apneic threshold is crossed, the signal to begin breathing increases, and if it is not too great, stable ventilation resumes after a short period of readjustment. However, if either the controller or the plant gain is too high, the loop gain will be greater than one, and the ventilatory response will overshoot, giving rise to hyperventilation and hypocapnia with or without arousal; hypopnea or apnea may subsequently result because of crossing the apneic threshold, and the pattern may be set up to repeat (Figure 10). This response sequence gives rise to periodic breathing, consisting of a series of repetitive central apneic events interspersed with a crescendo hyperpnea and subsequent hypopneic phase (Figure 11). Risk factors for this pattern include factors that increase controller gain, such as a low $PaCO_2$, a low FiO_2 (observed at altitude), or increased stimulation of afferents to the control center. When this periodic breathing pattern is accompanied by other clinical associations, central sleep apnea syndromes result.

Mixed Apneas

Occasionally, at the end of an otherwise predominantly central apnea, the resumption of the central signal occurs, but upper airway obstruction interferes with restoration of ventilation. This situation is termed a mixed apnea, and is depicted in Figures 12 and 13. Such events are similar to obstructive events in their associations with arousals and sleep fragmentation. However, mixed apneas may be more prevalent in patients with risk factors for central sleep apnea syndromes, such as congestive heart failure.

OBSTRUCTIVE SLEEP APNEA SYNDROME

Obstructive sleep apnea syndrome (OSAS) is currently defined by a combination of clinical factors and polygraphically measured factors. The most common accepted definitions of OSAS include an increased apnea-hypopnea index (the number of apneas plus hypopneas per hour of sleep) combined with symptoms or evidence of increased cardiovascular risk (Table 4). However, this definition must be regarded as a work in progress. Although it makes sense for the definition to include measures of observed breathing and sleep events, which events are most important: apneas, hypopneas, respiratory effort–related

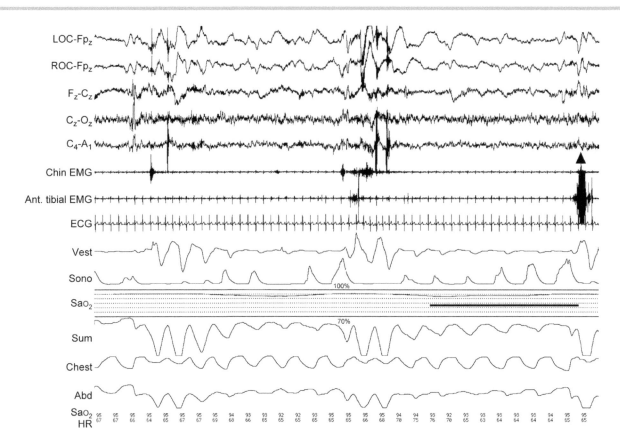

Figure 8 Respiratory Effort–Related Arousal. Bar shows period of increasing effort and decreasing flow, but no resulting significant desaturation. The event caused arousal (arrowhead), and lasted longer than 10 seconds, for a respiratory effort–related arousal. Note the crescendo of snore (Sono) volume and the thoracoabdominal paradox consistent with upper airway resistance. Vest indicates airflow from positive airway pressure pneumotachometer. For explanation of other labels, see Figure 5.

arousals, oxyhemoglobin desaturation events, overall arousals, or alterations in sleep architecture (e.g., the percentage of stage N1 in disease compared with normal)? Each of these variables has been studied with regard to the clinical manifestations of OSAS, and none of them seem closely correlated. For example, some studies show that cardiovascular risk correlates most closely with the frequency of oxygen desaturation from baseline, whereas sleepiness may correlate better with overall arousal index (5,8). The prevalence of an elevated apnea-hypopnea index (AHI) varies across age groups regardless of the presence or absence of sleep symptoms (Figure 14). For the present, the consensus definition of OSAS is an AHI ≥5 per hour with symptoms of sleepiness, cognitive difficulties, fatigue, or documented cardiovascular disease or hypertension, or an AHI ≥15 per hour even without symptoms (9).

OSAS is the most common of the sleep-related breathing disorders, with prevalence estimates of OSAS (when limited to persons with AHI ≥5 per hour and sleep symptoms) of 3% to 28%, with a prevalence of probably about 5% in Western countries (10). Independent risk factors for OSAS include age, increasing body mass index (BMI [weight in kg/height in m^2]), African American ethnicity, male sex, and pregnancy. Neck circumference is correlated with increased risk of OSAS, especially if exceeding 16.5 inches (40 cm) in men.

Clinical Presentation of Obstructive Sleep Apnea Syndrome

Sleep apnea syndromes are generally considered when a patient presents either with clinical symptoms of sleep apnea or clinical risk factors that are closely associated with sleep apnea. Once the patient is encountered, the clinical examination focuses on the elicitation of the symptoms of sleep-related breathing disorders and the identification of risk factors for either OSAS or central sleep apnea syndromes, concurrent cardiovascular risk factors, and factors that will influence treatment plans.

Symptoms, Associated Conditions, and Examination Findings
The clinical presentation of OSAS includes both daytime and nocturnal symptoms (Table 5). Disruptive snoring and excessive daytime sleepiness are most common, each being present in nearly 70% of patients (11). Various conditions have been associated with the increased prevalence of OSAS, chiefly due to the effect of associated craniofacial abnormalities or complex interactions of neuromuscular tone and anatomy (Table 6). Other diseases associated with a high prevalence of OSAS, but which may be complications of OSAS rather than causative factors, include hypertension, congestive heart failure, coronary artery disease, and stroke.

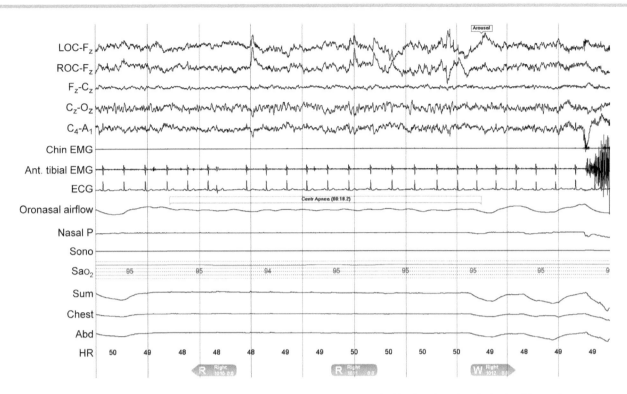

Figure 9 Central Apnea. The central apnea in this polysomnographic tracing is typical in that there is a lack of evidence for respiratory effort for 18.2 seconds. The lack of airflow is demonstrated both in the thermocouple (Oronasal airflow) and in the nasal pressure transducer. Resumption of breathing is gradual rather than abrupt. Central apneas during rapid eye movement (REM) sleep are less common than during non–rapid eye movement (NREM) sleep. Also unusual is the fact that arousals often occur after normal or even hyperpneic ventilation is achieved following central apnea, rather than at the onset of ventilation as shown here. This patient had Arnold-Chiari syndrome with frequent central apneas in both REM and NREM sleep. The electrocardiogram (ECG) shows an atrial premature contraction, but otherwise the patient is in sinus rhythm. For explanation of labels, see Figure 5.

During the physical examination, particular effort should be expended to examine the upper airway. In general, anatomical features that reduce upper airway patency when awake or at rest are correlated with an increased risk of OSAS (Table 7). Of these, the most practical and predictive seem to be the tongue position in relation to the soft palate, narrowing of the tonsillar pillars, tonsillar hypertrophy, tongue ridging, and neck circumference (12). The relationship between tongue position and the soft palate is conveniently summarized by the Friedman tongue position classification (also called the modified Mallampati scheme) as shown in Figure 15 (13). There is a good correlation between Friedman tongue position class and the prevalence of OSAS. In view of the similarity between the clinical symptoms of OSAS and Cheyne-Stokes breathing pattern (CSBP) or central sleep apnea, it is a good idea to also pay special attention during the cardiovascular examination to the possibility of atrial fibrillation or signs of left or right heart failure.

Before turning to diagnostic testing for OSAS, it is best to discuss the clinical presentation of a central sleep apnea syndrome, since many aspects are similar. The testing strategy should take into account both the likelihood of central sleep apnea syndrome and its probable treatment modalities.

CENTRAL SLEEP APNEA SYNDROMES

As shown in Table 1, there are six different types of central sleep apnea syndrome. By far the most common are CSBP, central sleep apnea secondary to stroke (medical conditions other than CSBP), and central sleep apnea due to chronic narcotic use.

Cheyne-Stokes Breathing Pattern

Central sleep apnea syndrome with CSBP (Figure 11) is common in patients with congestive heart failure, affecting 40% to 60% of such patients (14,15). Although the primary breathing events in this condition are repetitive centrally mediated apneas and hypopneas, snoring is also frequently present, as are witnessed apneas. Symptoms of CSBP are generally similar to those of patients with OSAS, except that insomnia, especially sleep-maintenance insomnia, appears to be more prevalent. Factors that are associated with an increased likelihood of having central rather than obstructive sleep apnea include the presence of atrial fibrillation, reduced left ventricular ejection fraction, male sex, and age older than 60 years (7). In slightly less than 20% of patients with CSBP and heart failure, periodic breathing may be observed during relaxed wakefulness in the

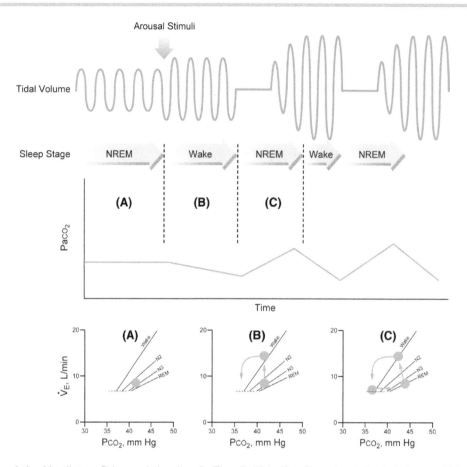

Figure 10 The Role of the Ventilatory Drive and the Apneic Threshold in the Genesis of Central Apnea. This sequence depicts a circumstance in which the sleeper begins with stable respiration but then experiences repetitive central apnea after arousal. (A [top and bottom panels]) At onset (far left), the patient is in stable stage N2 non–rapid eye movement (NREM) sleep. Tidal volume (top panel) is nearly constant; Pco$_2$ (lower 4-part panel) is constant at about 42 mm Hg. (B [top and bottom panels]) The patient experiences an arousal (cause not important) that rapidly moves the ventilatory control curve to the "Wake" line (bottom panel, B), and ventilation therefore increases (increased tidal volume and frequency, upper panel). If ventilatory drive is high, as may be seen in patients with congestive heart failure, for example, the Paco$_2$ will fall rapidly. In this example, Paco$_2$ falls to 36 mm Hg. (C [top and bottom panels]) The patient falls asleep, and the Paco$_2$ is below the apneic threshold of approximately 40 mm Hg. Therefore, there is no ventilatory drive until Paco$_2$ reaches 40 mm Hg, at which time ventilatory drive rises and ventilation begins again. If the ventilatory drive is high, the needed steady state ventilation may be overshot, producing an abrupt fall in Paco$_2$. In central apnea syndromes, an arousal often occurs coincident with the hyperpnea following the central apnea. Ventilatory control is again governed by the steeper wake curve (panel C), and as CO$_2$ falls and the patient returns to sleep, Paco$_2$ is again below the apneic threshold of 40 mm Hg, leading to repetitive cycling of central apneas interspersed with hyperpnea. REM indicates rapid eye movement; $\dot{V}_E$, minute ventilation.

daytime office encounter (16). Examination may disclose findings consistent with impaired left ventricular dysfunction, although patients often present for evaluation in a compensated condition. The presence of any of these risk factors, or the notable absence of risk factors associated with OSAS (e.g., increased BMI, increased neck circumference, or upper airway narrowing) should prompt consideration of CSBP.

Central Sleep Apnea Secondary to Stroke

Both central and obstructive sleep apneas are common and coexist in the setting of acute stroke, being present in more than 70% of patients in some reports. Over time, the prevalence of central sleep apnea events declines, with about 40% of patients found to have OSAS and fewer than 10% found to have central sleep apnea (17). In the acute situation, and occasionally in the

chronic case, central sleep apnea associated with stroke mimics the pattern seen in CSBP but with one notable exception: the period of the periodic cycles is much shorter in stroke than in CSBP associated with congestive heart failure (Figure 16) (17).

Symptoms are often dominated by those attributable to the stroke acutely, but later in the course of stroke, sleepiness that fails to resolve should prompt consideration of sleep apnea. Since both sleep apnea syndromes (i.e., obstructive and central) are associated with increased blood pressure and increased blood pressure lability, these factors should also prompt consideration of the diagnosis. There are many reasons to consider that treatment of either type of sleep apnea in patients with acute stroke might improve outcomes, including more favorable cardiovascular conditions, a reduction in circulating catecholamines, improved sleep quality, and a decrease in inflammatory markers. However, no studies to date show

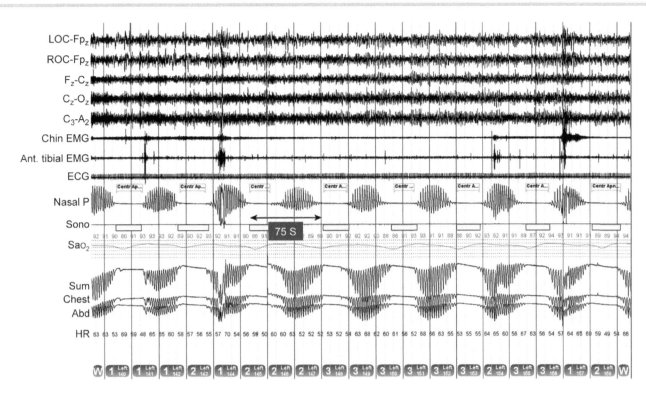

Figure 11 Periodic Breathing and Cheyne-Stokes Breathing. This polysomnographic tracing shows 600 seconds of non–rapid eye movement sleep with an apnea-hypopnea index of 69.2. The tracing demonstrates repetitive central apneas that are entered through a decrescendo breathing pattern and exited with a crescendo pattern. These apneas occur with mathematical periodicity; in this case the cycle time is 75 seconds (arrow), consistent with Cheyne-Stokes breathing, which is observed most often in patients with impaired heart failure, especially left ventricular dysfunction. Patients with acute stroke or who are not acclimated may also demonstrate periodic breathing patterns (with or without central apneas), but most often the cycle length is shorter, more on the order of 30 seconds. Current nosological efforts suggests that the diagnosis of Cheyne-Stokes breathing be reserved for cases in which the cycle length exceeds 45 seconds. Scrutiny of the electrocardiographic (ECG) tracing may reveal atrial fibrillation, a common accompaniment to Cheyne-Stokes breathing. For explanation of labels, see Figure 5.

unambiguously improved outcomes, and at least some studies show that positive airway pressure (PAP) therapy is poorly tolerated by many stroke patients.

Central Sleep Apnea Associated With Opiates

In recent years increased attention has focused on the management of patients with acute and chronic pain, and there has been a marked proliferation in chronic opiate use (Figure 17). Concomitantly, there is growing awareness that opiates are associated with central sleep apnea syndromes. For example, in a recent study of 98 patients using chronic opiates who were referred for suspected sleep-disordered breathing, 36% had OSAS, 24% had central sleep apnea syndrome, and 21% had a combination of obstructive and central sleep apneas (19). In contrast, most sleep disorders centers find that central sleep apnea syndrome is present in fewer than 5% of the patients referred to them for assessment. The proportion of central sleep apneas to obstructive sleep apneas in patients who use opiates appears to be dose dependent, with an increasing proportion of central apneas with higher doses of narcotics (Figure 18) (9,18,20).

Not only is central sleep apnea syndrome more common among opiate users but it also has characteristics that differ

from those of either CSBP or central sleep apnea secondary to stroke. The breathing pattern in opiate users frequently demonstrates an irregular ataxic pattern with central apneas randomly inserted throughout NREM sleep (Figure 19) (9,19,20). Other than a high prevalence and a somewhat unique pattern, the clinical presentation of opiate-related central sleep apnea syndrome does not appear substantially different from that of OSAS. However, this has not been systematically evaluated.

OTHER FORMS OF SLEEP-DISORDERED BREATHING

In addition to OSAS and central sleep apnea syndromes, which are mostly defined by discrete breathing events during sleep, there are primary sleep-related hypoventilatory disorders such as idiopathic sleep-related nonobstructive alveolar hypoventilation syndrome and congenital central alveolar hypoventilation syndrome (Table 1). In both of these disorders, intrinsic respiratory dysregulation leads to chronic hypoventilation with diurnal hypercapnia and, at times, to overt respiratory failure or sudden death. By far the most common causes of chronic sleep-related hypoventilation are obesity hypoventilation syndrome and hypoventilation due to neuromuscular or chest wall disorders.

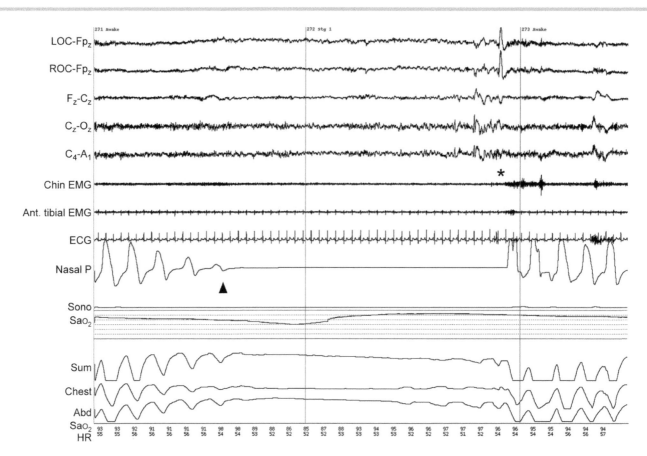

Figure 12 Mixed Apnea. In this polysomnographic tracing, the patient falls asleep and a sleep-onset central apnea ensues (see Figure 11). Resumption of ventilatory effort occurs but the upper airway is closed (arrowhead), and the apnea continues until an arousal (asterisk). Note the abrupt resumption of actual air movement, which is characteristic of an obstructive event. This event is a classic mixed apnea because it begins as a central event but ends as an obstructive one. For explanation of labels, see Figure 5.

Congenital central alveolar hypoventilation syndrome usually affects children, but it has also been reported in young adults (10). This unique sleep-related breathing disorder is associated with Hirschsprung disease and tumors of neural crest origin; in more than 90% of cases, it appears to result from a polyalanine repeat expansion mutation of the paired-like homobox 2b *(PHOX2B)* gene. Some investigators note that late-onset central alveolar hypoventilation syndrome may involve other mutations of the *PHOX2B* gene. There is considerable debate as to whether congenital central alveolar hypoventilation syndrome and late-onset central alveolar hypoventilation syndrome are separate disease entities or merely parts of a spectrum of congenital alveolar hypoventilation syndrome. In addition, since the genetic mutations involved in alveolar hypoventilation were discovered relatively recently, some speculative reports on adults with idiopathic central alveolar hypoventilation syndrome construe it as perhaps instead being due to *PHOX2B* mutations (10,21).

Congenital central alveolar hypoventilation syndrome typically presents in an otherwise normal-appearing infant noted to breathe radically or only very shallowly during sleep. A diligent search reveals no endocrine, cardiac, pulmonary, or neuromuscular causation. Infants who present at birth often require intubation and mechanically assisted ventilation.

Other infants may appear to breathe adequately, while awake or when being examined clinically, but they also have abrupt intervals of hypoventilation with hypoxemia and hypercapnia that are noted typically when they sleep or occasionally when they are awake. Clinical findings may be noted as cyanosis, an apparent life-threatening event, right heart failure, or even hypoxic neurological damage. In infancy, congenital central alveolar hypoventilation syndrome is a severe disease, most often requiring diurnal ventilatory support. Hirschsprung disease is noted in approximately 16% of cases, and neural tumors such as ganglioneuromas or ganglioneuroblastomas, swallowing dysfunction, strabismus, or other autonomic dysfunction may be present. Irregular breathing patterns, apnea, edema, and lethargy are presenting features. Notably, when hypoxic, these children do not show clinically significant signs of respiratory distress, such as retractions or nasal flaring. Therefore, significant gas exchange abnormalities may be present over long periods of time without detection. Because the severity of hypoventilation varies, upper respiratory tract infections, diarrhea, or other causes of fever may precipitate bouts of respiratory failure.

Late-onset central alveolar hypoventilation syndrome is characterized by sequelae of hypoventilation, such as morning headache, polycythemia, poorly refreshing sleep, daytime

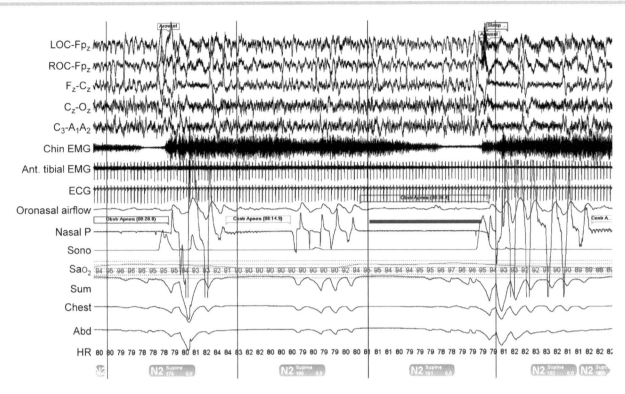

Figure 13 Central and Mixed Apneas. This figure depicts 120 seconds of stage N2 sleep that is interrupted by four ventilatory events. Focusing on the second marked event, we recognize a central apnea lasting 14.9 seconds. There is a lack of perceivable respiratory effort (no movement in the chest [Chest] or abdominal [Abd] respiratory inductance plethysmography bands), and at the beginning of the apnea there are fine oscillations in the nasal pressure (Nasal P) and oronasal airflow thermocouple tracings coincident with cardiac contractions (cardioballistographic tracings). Following recovery breaths, there is again the onset of a central apnea, but this time it is accompanied by the onset of efforts to breathe during the terminal 5 seconds of the apnea. Apneas that contain such central and obstructive components are called *mixed apneas.* Because these contain an obstructive component, some guidelines have suggested that they be counted along with other purely obstructive events (here the event is labeled an obstructive apnea, although it is actually a mixed apnea). Since the genesis of mixed apneas may be quite different from purely obstructive events, one might expect this practice to change in the coming years. For explanation of labels, see Figure 5.

Table 4 Diagnostic criteria for obstructive sleep apnea syndrome

Clinical factors	Polysomnographic factors
Complains of unintentional sleep episodes during wakefulness, daytime sleepiness, unrefreshing sleep, fatigue, or insomnia Self-reported breath holding, gasping, or choking upon awakening Witnessed loud snoring, breathing interruptions, or both	Apneas plus hypopneas plus RERAs occur ≥5 times per hour of sleep. These events are assumed to be predominantly consistent with obstructive events.[a]
Cardiovascular disease, such as hypertension, coronary artery disease, or stroke	Data indicate increased cardiovascular events in untreated patients with AHI ≥5 per hour of sleep. Treatment is therefore often advised with AHI ≥5 and existing cardiovascular disease, even without significant symptoms, and third-party payers often supplement the cost of therapy. These events are assumed to be predominantly consistent with obstructive events.
None required	Apneas plus hypopneas plus RERAs occur ≥15 times per hour of sleep.[a] For many insurance companies, only apneas and hypopneas are considered, so AHI ≥15 will suffice.

Abbreviations: AHI, apnea-hypopnea index; RERA, respiratory effort–related arousal.
[a]AASM. The International Classification of Sleep Disorders: Diagnostic and Coding Manual. 2nd ed. Westchester (IL): American Academy of Sleep Medicine, 2005.

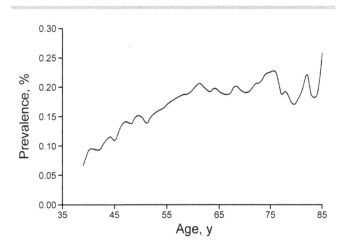

Figure 14   Age and Prevalence of Sleep-Disordered Breathing. The prevalence of sleep-disordered breathing with an apnea-hypopnea index of >15 increases with aging until about age 60 years. (From Young T, Shahar E, Nieto FJ, et al; Sleep Heart Health Study Research Group. Predictors of sleep-disordered breathing in community-dwelling adults: the Sleep Heart Health Study. Arch Intern Med 2002; 162:893-900. [Used with permission.])

Table 6   Conditions associated with increased risk of obstructive sleep apnea syndrome

Conditions
Acromegaly
Alcohol use
Arnold-Chiari malformation
Congestive heart failure
Coronary artery disease
Crouzon disease
Cushing syndrome (exogenous or endogenous)
Heart transplantation
Hypertension
Klippel-Feil syndrome
Myxedema
Obesity
Pierre Robin syndrome
Postpolio syndrome
Prader-Willi syndrome
Stroke
Trisomy 21

Table 5   Symptoms of obstructive sleep apnea syndrome

Daytime symptoms	Nocturnal symptoms
Sleepiness	Snoring
Morning headaches	Witnessed apneas
Poor concentration	Choking spells
Cognitive dysfunction	Restless sleep
Personality changes	Insomnia
Erectile dysfunction in men	Nocturia
Lower-extremity edema	Diaphoresis
	Reflux
	Drooling
	Moaning

Table 7   Features on examination associated with obstructive sleep apnea syndrome

Features
Obesity
Increased neck circumference
Nasal obstruction
Retrognathia
Overjet
Enlarged tongue (dental ridging on lateral aspects may indicate that tongue is too large for existing space)
High-arched palate
Tonsillar hypertrophy
Narrowing of the tonsillar pillars
Elongation or enlargement of the uvula

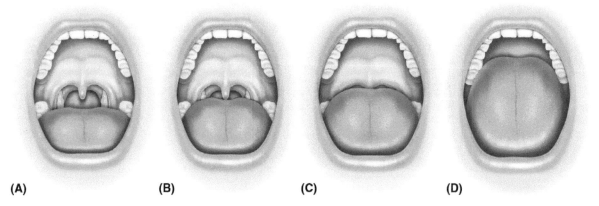

(A)   **(B)**   **(C)**   **(D)**

Figure 15   Friedman Tongue Position Classification (Modified Mallampati Scheme). During the physical examination, the patient is asked to open the mouth widely with the tongue left in place. Oropharyngeal crowding is graded as follows: (A) Grade 1: tonsils, pillars, and soft palate are clearly visible; (B) grade 2: only the uvula, pillars, and upper pole are visible; (C) grade 3: only part of the soft palate is visible, and the tonsils, pillars, and tip of the uvula cannot be seen; or (D) grade 4: only the hard palate is visible and not even the arches on either side of the uvula can be seen. Using this scheme rather than adjectives such as "crowded oropharynx" results in clearer communication and greater reproducibility among examiners about the degree of airway crowding. (Adapted from Friedman et al [13]. [Used witih permission.])

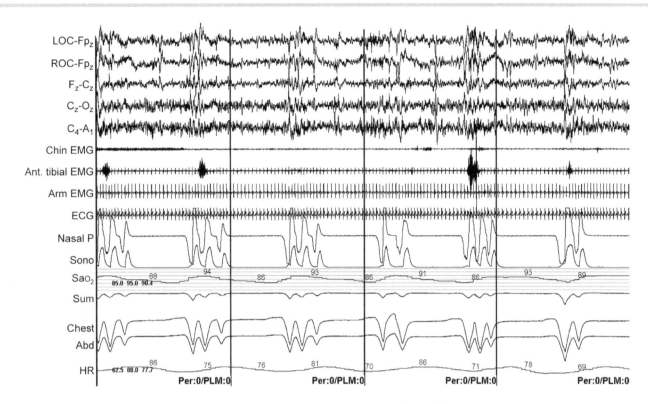

Figure 16 Periodic Breathing in Stroke. In contrast to the long cycle time seen in Cheyne-Stokes breathing, this tracing, obtained from a patient shortly after a left hemispheric stroke, shows an apnea-hypopnea index of 23 that is composed almost exclusively of repetitive central apneas marching in a periodic fashion with a short cycle time of less than 30 seconds. Continuous positive airway pressure is usually highly ineffective for this pattern, and it was poorly tolerated by the patient. For explanation of labels, see Figure 5.

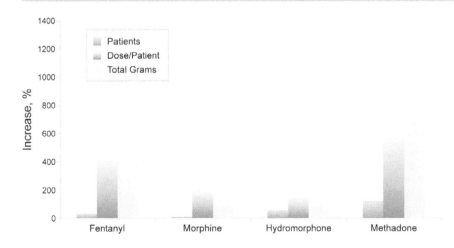

Figure 17 Percentage Increases in Use of Prescription Narcotics (1997–2006). Over about a decade in which there was increased treatment of chronic pain, there was a doubling in the number of patients for whom narcotics were prescribed and increases in the number of prescribed narcotic doses per patient. Thus, the total grams prescribed annually also increased substantially. It is therefore likely that physicians treating patients with sleep apnea will encounter patients who are chronic users of high-dose opiates. (From Morgenthaler [18]. [Used with permission.])

sleepiness, pulmonary hypertension, peripheral edema, or cor pulmonale. Ventilatory studies demonstrate decreased hypercapnic and hypoxic ventilatory drive during both wakefulness and sleep. During polysomnography, decreased tidal volume may last many minutes, and the patient may experience sustained severe arterial oxygen desaturation. Perhaps somewhat counterintuitively, the episodes worsen during REM sleep,

which would not be expected in a defect of chemosensitivity ventilatory regulation because such defects typically manifest primarily during NREM sleep.

For many neuromuscular disorders, ventilatory insufficiency is life limiting. In nearly all cases, ventilatory insufficiency is most severe during sleep. For example, in amyotrophic lateral sclerosis, diaphragm strength is often

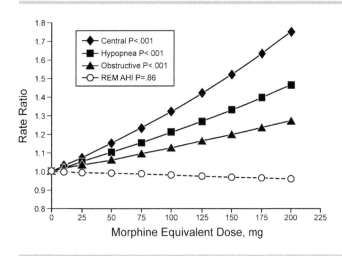

Figure 18   Rate of Apneas as a Function of Opioid Dose. The rate ratio for the development of central apneas, hypopneas, obstructive apneas, and apnea-hypopnea index (AHI) during rapid eye movement (REM) sleep was explored as a function of morphine equivalent doses in a population of chronic opiate users referred to a sleep center compared with patients not using opioids who were referred to the same center and matched by sex, age, and body mass index. In all cases, narcotic dose significantly affected the frequency of these events compared with those in nonusers. (From Walker et al [9]. [Used with permission.])

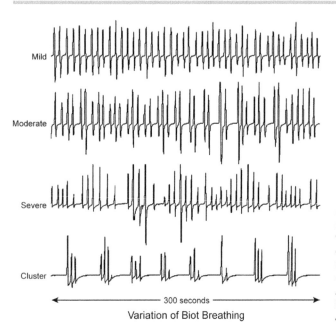

Figure 19   Irregular Breathing Pattern in Chronic Opiate Users. Not only is the frequency of central apneas increased with opiate use but also the ventilatory pattern becomes more irregular, or ataxic. Various gradations of ataxic breathing patterns occur in chronic opiate users, ranging from mild ataxia, to Biot breathing as seen here, to cluster breathing pattern. (From Farney RJ, Walker JM, Boyle KM, Cloward TV, Shilling KC. Adaptive servoventilation [ASV] in patients with sleep disordered breathing associated with chronic opioid medications for non-malignant pain. J Clin Sleep Med 2008; 4:311-9. [Used with permission.])

reduced disproportionately to axial muscles. In these cases, the atonia associated with normal REM sleep provides a severe challenge to ventilation because the patient is dependent upon diaphragm function at that time. The result is deep oxyhemoglobin desaturation, hypercapnia, and deteriorating sleep quality. The presentation consists of both ventilatory and sleep-related abnormalities. A gradual reduction in baseline oxygen saturation, increased diurnal Pco_2, decreased vital capacity, and decreased inspiratory muscle strength are accompanied by a decline in the quality of sleep. Patients may begin to notice orthopnea and headaches on awakening.

DIAGNOSIS OF SLEEP-RELATED BREATHING DISORDERS

All sleep-related breathing disorders may be diagnosed with polysomnography. A patient suspected of having a sleep-related breathing disorder on the basis of a clinical presentation

or risk factors should be considered for polysomnography. When OSAS is thought likely and the patient has no concurrent risk factors for central sleep apnea syndrome or central alveolar hypoventilation syndromes, a portable cardiopulmonary monitor may prove sufficient (see chapter 5). In situations with considerable risk of central sleep apnea syndrome or alveolar hypoventilation syndromes, polysomnography is the test of choice.

Obstructive Sleep Apnea Syndrome

The diagnosis of OSAS requires a combination of clinical and polysomnographic findings. In the presence of clinical findings as described above, five or more respiratory events (obstructive apneas, hypopneas, or respiratory effort–related arousals) per hour of sleep are sufficient to diagnose OSAS. Some patients have little or no discernible clinical symptoms. In these cases, 15 or more respiratory events per hour of sleep are sufficient to diagnose OSAS. A severity grading system has been suggested: mild obstructive sleep apnea (AHI 5-15), moderate obstructive sleep apnea (AHI 15-30), and severe obstructive sleep apnea (AHI $\geq$30). Of course, this scheme does not take into account the severity of oxyhemoglobin desaturation or of sleepiness experienced by the patient. Some patients with a relatively mild AHI experience severe daytime hypersomnolence that corrects or improves with therapy, and vice versa. The diagnostic criteria for pediatric OSAS are in a state of flux, but generally symptoms combined with more than one scorable respiratory event per hour and polysomnographic evidence of an association of arousals or gas exchange abnormalities related to upper airway obstruction are sufficient for diagnosis.

Central Sleep Apnea Syndrome
Central sleep apnea syndrome is said to be present when there are five or more central apneas per hour of sleep. Because central and obstructive events often coexist in a given patient, many clinicians diagnose central sleep apnea syndrome when the central apnea index is greater than or equal to five AND the total central apnea index is greater than or equal to 50% of the total number of respiratory events. CSBP has historically been described by the visual recognition of the waxing and waning ventilatory pattern in the appropriate clinical setting. In the recently published ICSD-2 (*International Classification of Sleep Disorders*, 2nd edition) (22), it has been suggested that polysomnography shows at least 10 central apneas and hypopneas per hour of sleep with the hypopneas demonstrating the crescendo-decrescendo pattern and frequent arousals from sleep. Other scoring schemes try to impose measures of either the duration or percentage of CSBP, as noted, but there is little agreement in this regard. The central periodic breathing pattern associated with stroke is considered to be a subset of central sleep apnea syndrome or periodic breathing, and it is identified by a central apnea index of five or more associated with a short crescendo-decrescendo ventilatory pattern.

Central Alveolar Hypoventilation Syndrome
The polysomnographic diagnosis of central alveolar hypoventilation syndrome requires episodes of shallow breathing or apneas longer than 10 seconds combined with oxyhemoglobin desaturation and frequent arousals and/or heart rate variability as a result of these breathing abnormalities. Observed apneas should be central, and hypopneas should not show signs of increased upper airway resistance. In a literal sense, an increase in $Paco_2$ of at least 10 mm Hg should be demonstrated as a result of sleep. However, current technology does not provide a very reliable means of measuring this directly; its measurement is generally reserved for research settings. Clinical measurements of $Paco_2$ may be estimated by using transcutaneous CO_2 or end-tidal CO_2 sensors. By definition, patients with these syndromes ought to demonstrate diurnal hypercapnia by an arterial blood gas showing a $Paco_2$ greater than 45 mm Hg.

TREATMENT OF OBSTRUCTIVE SLEEP APNEA SYNDROMES
OSAS is a chronic medical condition that requires proper diagnosis, a comprehensive treatment plan, and long-term follow-up (Table 8). It is important to note that the mortality associated with OSAS is predominantly due to cardiovascular disease; thus, the comprehensive care of these patients should ensure that such issues are addressed in concert with OSAS.

Chronic diseases are best managed by enlisting patients in self-care. Therapy for OSAS begins with educating the patient about the disease. Patients should be taught how it affects their health and quality of life, with an emphasis on the fact that leaving it untreated puts them at increased risk for motor vehicle accidents, possible cognitive and mood disturbances, and an increased likelihood of experiencing cardiovascular events. Patients should avoid driving when drowsy and, in the case of professional drivers and pilots, should be aware that their licensing and employment may require proof that therapy is adequate.

Lifestyle
Lifestyle factors that contribute to airway collapse include alcohol ingestion and obesity, so patients should be counseled to avoid alcohol close to bedtime and should be encouraged to obtain a healthy weight. In some patients, these efforts alone may suffice to treat their OSAS. Weight loss is fairly reliably associated with improvement in airway patency. In some studies, as many as 30% of patients achieve a cure (23). Unfortunately, achieving adequate weight loss is difficult and takes time, so moderate to severe OSAS requires careful monitoring and definitive treatment in the interim. Furthermore, some patients who maintain their weight loss will still experience a worsening of their OSAS. The reasons for this have not been systematically investigated, but it may be that fat redistribution or adaptation in neuromuscular control over time adversely affects airway patency during sleep. Additional attention should be focused on addressing ways to improve sleep hygiene and ensure adequate total sleep duration.

Positional Therapy
Changing from a supine sleeping posture may be a successful positional therapy for some patients, especially if they have demonstrated mild to moderate OSAS with a largely positional component. Positional therapy should not be recommended for persons who cannot maintain a side sleeping posture due to orthopedic- or pain-related problems. Positional therapy may be initiated by using feedback devices that prompt side sleeping postures (Figure 20). Long-term adherence to these therapies is incompletely understood. One survey found that only about 30% of patients were adherent to positional recommendations after a year, with the most common reason for discontinuation being pain or discomfort (24).

Oral Appliances
The most common oral appliance used in the management of OSAS is the mandibular advancement device (MAD) (Figure 21) (25,26). It mechanically protrudes the mandible. Although protrusion of the mandible might be expected to enhance airway patency predominantly by increasing the anteroposterior airway dimension, this has not proved to be the case. Instead, studies using magnetic resonance imaging before and after the fitting of a MAD show that the improvement occurs predominantly in the lateral dimension. These devices, when properly fitted and adjusted, lead to a 50% improvement in AHI in about 65% of patients and to cure (AHI <5) in about 35% to 40% of patients (27). Patients with mild or moderate obstructive sleep apnea are the most suitable for MAD

Table 8   Management of obstructive sleep apnea syndrome

Phase	Suggested time	Objectives	Tools
Preventive care	Periodic health examinations; engagement of health care system	Prevent development of obstructive sleep apnea Detect presence of risk factors for obstructive sleep apnea so that health care system may be activated toward detection, if indicated	Promotion of healthy lifestyles; ideal body weight Screening questionnaires for sleep apnea Pointed questioning of patients with strong risk factors
Diagnosis	When disease is suspected	Obtain accurate diagnosis of suspected sleep disorder	Polysomnography Portable monitors
Initial care plan formulation	As soon as diagnosis is confirmed	Integrate evidence-based practice with patient preferences and constraints to decide on best treatment modalities Consider multiple issues that require attention (airway, lifestyles, comorbidities such as cardiovascular disease, diabetes, obesity, hypertension)	Positional therapy Oral appliances Positive airway pressure Surgical modification of the upper airway Weight loss and management Cardiovascular primary and secondary prevention Management of diabetes (primary or referral) Lifestyle modification (tobacco, alcohol, caffeine) Sleep hygiene improvement
Initial follow-up care	1 Day to 4 weeks after initiation of treatment plan	Assessment of efficacy of initial care plan Reinforcement of initial care plan interventions and education Reformulation of plans based on open and active listening and assessment Assure proper function of technology such as PAP machines, masks, humidifiers, and oral appliances	Interview Sleepiness assessment (Epworth Sleepiness Scale, visual analog scales, quality-of-life assessment) Direct visual inspection of equipment; observation of patient on equipment at treatment pressure Downloading of PAP compliance and effectiveness data Overnight oximetry or portable monitoring, if needed
Longitudinal management	Every 6 to 12 months	Prevent complications of obstructive sleep apnea Address any side effects of therapy Ensure ongoing effectiveness of therapy plan Adapt plans to changing health and social status of patient	Periodic follow-up visits with interview and examination Reassessment of comorbidities such as cardiovascular disease, hypertension, diabetes control, and weight management or referral as appropriate Sleepiness assessment (Epworth Sleepiness Scale, visual analog scale, quality-of-life assessment) Direct visual inspection of equipment; observation of patient on equipment at treatment pressure Downloading of PAP compliance and effectiveness data Overnight oximetry or portable monitoring

Abbreviation: PAP, positive airway pressure.

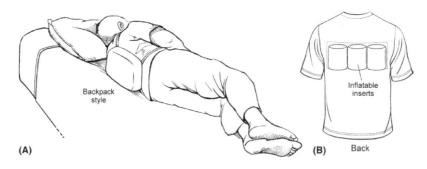

(A)   Backpack style

(B)   Inflatable inserts   Back

Figure 20   Positional Therapy Devices. The most common positional therapy assist devices make sleeping supine uncomfortable or impossible. These range in level of complexity from simple "tennis-ball-in-a-T-shirt" devices to complex strap-on backpack-like devices. Not pictured, and not truly tested for sleep apnea, are electronic devices that issue chirps or alarms when the sleeper moves to the supine position. Special pillows also may attempt to optimize head position, but these have shown only modest improvement at best in the apnea-hypopnea index of patients with obstructive sleep apnea.

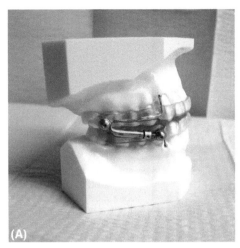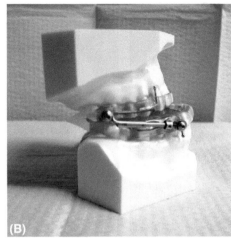

Figure 21 Mandibular Advancement Device for Treatment of Obstructive Sleep Apnea. The mandibular advancement device is the most common type of oral appliance for treating patients with obstructive sleep apnea. The one pictured here is a titratable device. (A) There is minimal protrusion of the mandible early in treatment. (B) Over time, the protrusion may be lengthened to the extent of the patient's tolerance or of the device's effectiveness.

Table 9 Complications of oral appliances used for treatment of obstructive sleep apnea syndrome

Complication or side effect	Frequency, %[a]
Gagging	10
Temporary or permanent occlusive change	6–12
Gum pain	9–40
Muscle or myofascial pain	10–40
Excessive salivation	20–30
Dry mouth	23–30
Dental discomfort or pain	26–60
Temporomandibular joint pain	26
Unable to wear	10–30

[a] Ferguson KA, Cartwright R, Rogers R, Schmidt-Nowara W. Oral appliances for snoring and obstructive sleep apnea: a review. Sleep 2006; 29:244-62.

treatment. Positional improvement in the AHI in the lateral position and lower BMI are predictive of a better response. MADs may be used only in patients with an adequate number of healthy teeth in each dental arch (usually eight) and can lead to complications (Table 9). Although PAP is uniformly more successful in reducing the AHI and improving sleepiness, some patients adhere better to a MAD. Therefore, in patients without contraindications and with favorable prognostic indicators, a MAD should be offered as a therapy choice. When immediate or certain improvement in OSAS is needed, continuous positive airway pressure (CPAP) should be considered first.

Positive Airway Pressure Therapy

PAP therapy provides a pneumatic splint to the upper airway. Airway pressure sufficient to open the airway enough to eliminate airflow limitations to breathing does so by increasing the retropharyngeal space in the lateral dimension more so than in the anteroposterior dimension (Figures 22 and 23). The components of a PAP device are shown in Figure 24. There is a wide variety of such devices available to enhance patient comfort or

address specific breathing disorders. By far the most common modality is CPAP. The treatment pressure for CPAP is most reliably determined by adjusting the pressure during attended polysomnography until the sleep-disordered breathing events have stopped. Because obstructive events are more common in stage REM sleep and when supine, optimal CPAP titration requires that the treatment pressure be observed during polysomnography in REM sleep while the patient is supine (28). In select patients with moderate to severe OSAS and no complicating medical conditions, automatic titrating PAP devices may be used either as primary therapy or as a temporary treatment to determine a fixed pressure for ongoing therapy with a CPAP device (Figure 25). The optimal time over which an automatic titrating PAP device must gather data in order to estimate the CPAP treatment is not known, but it is typically a period of at least two weeks of compliant use.

PAP is foreign to every patient initially, and its proper introduction is essential to long-term success in CPAP therapy. There are no studies evaluating the impact of prepolysomnographic patient education, but nearly all patients and sleep laboratories can testify to the benefits of educating the patient about OSAS and CPAP therapy, and of introducing and fitting CPAP before the sleep study. At our facility, patients are allowed to sit with a CPAP device on at low pressures before the study. This allows adjustments to fit, and if needed, desensitization to the apparatus. Such an approach also seems prudent before sending a PAP-naïve patient home with an automatic titrating PAP device.

The interface fit and comfort cannot be overemphasized. Fortunately, there are a wide variety of interface types and sizes, some of which may be seen in Figure 26. In addition to careful mask fitting, other ways to improve patient comfort include use of a heated humidity chamber (especially when the patient has underlying nasal or sinus symptoms, uses drying medications, or lives in a dry or cool climate), pressure-contouring devices (Figure 27), or special pillows that assist in maintaining a comfortable position while using a PAP device (29).

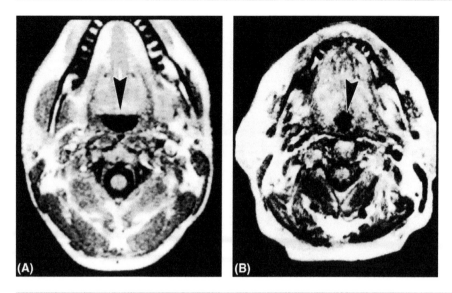

Figure 22 Upper Airway Dimensions in Obstructive Sleep Apnea. Magnetic resonance imaging scans show transverse sections of the pharynx (arrowhead) in (A) a subject without obstructive sleep apnea compared to (B) a subject with obstructive sleep apnea. Note that, compared with that of the subject without obstructive sleep apnea, the lateral dimension of the pharynx is decreased more so than the anteroposterior dimension. (From Ryan CM, Bradley TD. Pathogenesis of obstructive sleep apnea. J Appl Physiol 2005; 99:2440-50. [Used with permission.])

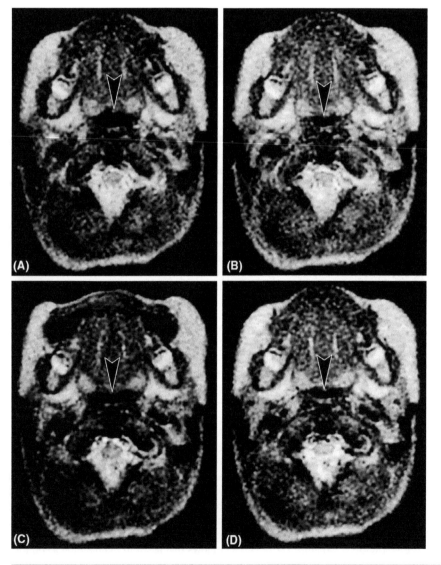

Figure 23 Effects of Continuous Positive Airway Pressure on Upper Airway Dimensions. Magnetic resonance imaging scans of the airway (arrowhead) of this subject under light propofol sedation reveal (A) a resemblance to the normal airway observed in Figure 22A. (B) With deeper propofol anesthesia, the airway more closely resembles that of a patient with obstructive sleep apnea (OSA) as seen in Figure 22B. (C) When continuous positive airway pressure (CPAP) of 10 cm H_2O is applied, the lateral dimensions of the airway increase dramatically. (D) With removal of CPAP and deepening of propofol anesthesia, the airway returns to a more collapsed configuration like that of a patient with OSA. Other studies have also shown that CPAP seems to increase the lateral dimension of the airway more so than it does the anteroposterior position. Similarly, the lateral walls of the pharynx appear more collapsible in patients with OSA. (From Crawford MW, Rohan D, Macgowan CK, Yoo S-J, Macpherson BA. Effect of propofol anesthesia and continous positive airway pressure on upper airway size and configuration in infants. Anesthesiology 2006; 105:45-50. [Used with permission.])

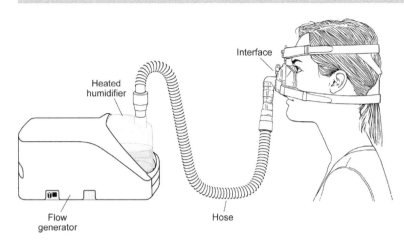

Figure 24 Components of Positive Airway Pressure Therapy. The basic components of positive airway pressure therapy for treatment of obstructive sleep apnea include a flow generator that produces pressurized air. The pressure may be continuous positive airway pressure (CPAP) or other pressure designed to best address the patient's underlying problem. Different flow generators may deliver pressure with expiratory pressure relief, bilevel pressure, automatically titrating pressure, variable pressure contours, or adaptive pressure levels with or without contours. For enhanced comfort and compliance, the air should be warmed and humidified (heated humidity chamber). In modern designs, the humidity chamber is often directly attached to the flow generator and the pressurized air passes through the humidifier before passing through the hose (or tubing) to the interface. Numerous interfaces, such as the nasal mask pictured here, are available to help provide a seal with the patient's airway.

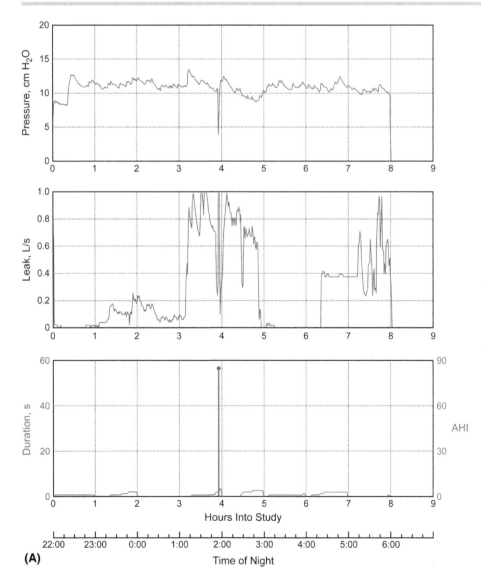

(A)

Figure 25 Autotitrating Positive Airway Pressure. (A) These data were downloaded from an autotitrating positive airway pressure device used to treat patients with moderately severe obstructive sleep apnea. The bottom panel shows a running tally of apneas and hypopneas detected by the machine over time. In the top panel, the delivered pressure is constantly being adjusted to the conditions being detected. When there is a lack of events, the pressure tends downward to 10 to 11 cm H_2O. However, when the device detects events, it increases pressure in an attempt to eliminate them. During this particular night, the pressure varied from 7 cm H_2O to 13 cm H_2O. Note that in the middle of the night there was a marked increase in estimated mask leak. Such leaks make the estimate of respiratory events less sensitive and less specific. If high leak is an ongoing or common problem, the patient may find continuous positive airway pressure uncomfortable and/or ineffective. AHI indicates apnea-hypopnea index. (*Continued next page.*)

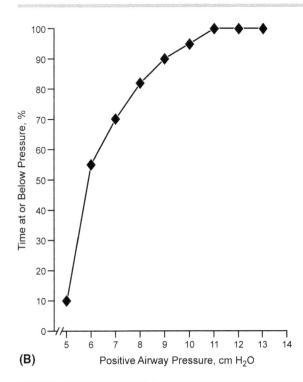

(B)

Figure 25 Continued (B) The data from many such nights may be tabulated to develop a cumulative distribution of pressures. These data were taken at 2 months of use. They show that 90% of the time, the estimated needed pressure is ≤9 cm H_2O, whereas 95% of the time the needed pressure appears to be ≤10 cm H_2O. A reasonable choice for a fixed pressure for ongoing treatment might be 10 cm H_2O.

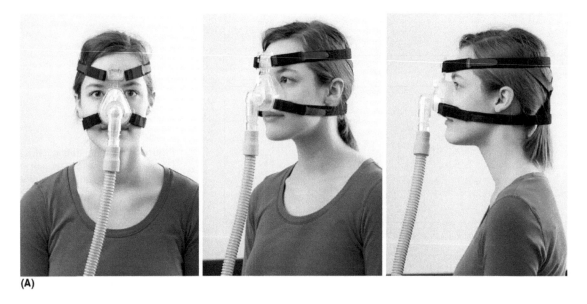

(A)

Figure 26 Types of Positive Airway Pressure Interfaces. (A) The nasal mask is among the most common of the interfaces used in positive airway pressure therapy. It fits over the nose, does not cover the mouth, and is highly stable over the face. It distributes pressure over a large area and can be tightened when high pressures are needed without inducing too much discomfort. (B) Nasal pillows are also favorites of patients. Since these interfaces have a lower profile and footprint on the face, some studies show a reduced sense of claustrophobia and enhanced compliance with them compared with nasal masks. Because the contact area is small, the interfaces may become dislodged or not seal well at higher pressures or when the patient rolls to one side. Tightening the mask to improve the seal may result in too much pressure for comfort. (C) Oronasal, or "full face" masks, cover both the nasal and oral airways. This type of mask may be necessary when the patient has a great deal of mouth leak or when the patient prefers the fit. These are not our usual first choice for patients with obstructive sleep apnea, but they are often used to provide noninvasive positive airway pressure ventilation. (D) The hybrid interface combines nasal pillows with an oral airway. It may work for patients who have significant mouth leak problems but do not want the bulk of an oronasal mask. This type of mask covers little of the area over or near the eyes, so may induce less claustrophobia in those requiring a mouth seal.

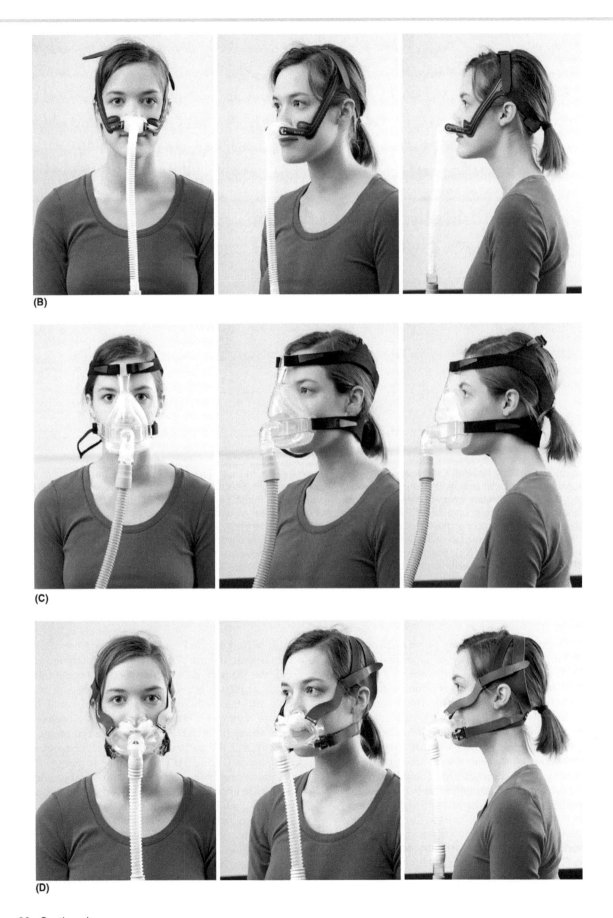

(B)

(C)

(D)

Figure 26 Continued

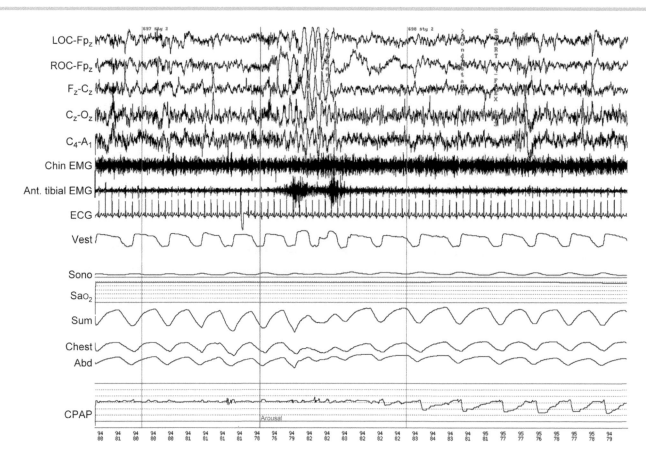

Figure 27 Expiratory Pressure Relief in Otherwise Continuous Positive Airway Pressure Therapy. Sometimes patients have a heightened sensitivity to pressure that is particularly evident during exhalation against pressure. Some flow generators automatically reduce the pressure when they detect the exhaled breath, which is called expiratory pressure relief. In this polysomnographic tracing, the patient is in stage N2 sleep with continuous positive airway pressure (CPAP) of 12 cm H_2O. The arousal (vertical red line) occurs without definite cause, although the flattening of the inspiratory contour on the flow channel (Vest) suggests that there may yet be some residual obstruction despite the CPAP of 12 cm H_2O. The technologist elects to set the C-Flex (Philips Respironics, Inc, Andover, Massachusetts) at the least resistant setting of 3 (just after the second epoch of stage N2). The CPAP contour (bottom tracing) shows a transient reduction of pressure of about 3 cm H_2O with each exhale. CPAP with expiratory pressure relief has been shown to be as effective as CPAP without expiratory pressure relief, and in some cases it may even enhance patient comfort. Vest indicates airflow as measured by positive airway pressure pneumotachometer. For explanation of other labels, see Figure 5.

Despite these measures, PAP may prove difficult for the patient to use. Long-term compliance is determined to some extent by early experiences with PAP, often within a week or so of initiation. Because of this, follow-up is recommended within 1 to 4 weeks after initiating PAP therapy. The follow-up visit should focus clinically on any comfort issues, on whether snoring is noted during use (an indicator of inadequate pressure to control obstruction), and on whether there has been subjective improvement in sleepiness or other pretreatment symptoms. Additionally, downloaded compliance reports may produce much useful information about the degree of leak and the patterns and regularity of use (Figures 28 and 29).

Surgical Modifications of the Airway for Obstructive Sleep Apnea Syndrome

Surgical interventions primarily focus on increasing the dimension and tone of the oropharynx. The most common types of surgical procedures are the uvulopalatopharyngoplasty, the genioglossus advancement and hyoid myotomy, the modified

hyoid myotomy and suspension, and maxillomandibular advancement (Figure 30). After a rhinolaryngoscopy assessment, the primary sites of obstruction are determined and a surgical approach is chosen to address the site of obstruction (Table 10). Successful surgical therapies would be desirable because they will ensure adherence. However, although improvement in the AHI and subjective symptoms is observed in nearly half the patients who are treated surgically, cure is less common (Figure 31) (30). Because surgery is more expensive, has higher risks, and is less predictably effective, most patients are encouraged to try PAP or an oral appliance before considering surgery. Exceptions to this conservative approach would be children or young adults with notable adenotonsillar hypertrophy, for whom a surgical approach is often the initial treatment. Even in these cases, cure rates are often not as good as hoped and patients should undergo follow-up evaluation with home sleep testing or polysomnography.

The results with maxillomandibular advancement have been a bit more encouraging, with objective treatment success rates typically greater than 80% when the treatment is provided

Summary of Compliance: All Data

Compliance Statistics

Date range (days)	11/19/2008-8/30/2009 (285 days)
Days with device usage	151 days
Days without device usage	134 days
Percentage of days with device usage	53%
Cumulative usage	844 h 34 min
Maximum usage (1 day)	8 h 47 min
Average usage (all days)	2 h 58 min
Average usage (days used)	5 h 36 min
Minimum usage (1 day)	28 min
Percentage of days with usage ≥4 hours	43.5%
Percentage of days with usage <4 hours	56.5%

CPAP Compliance (11/19/2008-8/30/2009)

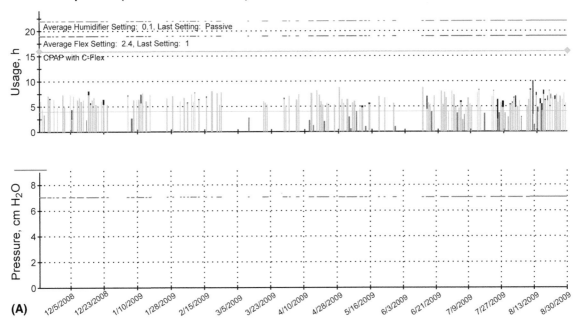

(A)

Figure 28 Positive Airway Pressure Compliance Reports. (A) Actual compliance data from November 19, 2008, to August 30, 2009, in a patient with severe obstructive sleep apnea (apnea-hypopnea index, 46): (Top) Summary of all compliance data, and (Bottom) hours of usage and pressure readings over time. A previously highly successful and compliant user of continuous positive airway pressure (CPAP) had a follow-up visit on August 7, 2009, and reported good usage and improvement in symptoms, with a reduction in her Epworth Sleepiness Scale score from 16 to 7. However, a review of the compliance data showed actual usage of the CPAP device on only 53% of all days, and the patient admitted that she "just got sick of it" sometimes and had not used it on those nights. She had several other health problems, including a recent kidney transplant, hypertension, diabetes mellitus, and obesity, and she was also struggling with depression. Inspection of the system showed an open oxygen port that had been attached during a hospitalization in March 2009. Removal of the oxygen port returned leakage to the normal range. Mask comfort was readdressed, and the patient was shown how to use the heated humidity (left turned off before this visit). A return visit was scheduled for August 30, 2009. (B, see next page) At that time, the patient showed an improved pattern of CPAP use (daily use from 08/14/09 to 08/30/09). She still had not turned on the heated humidity and had to be reminded about how to do so. At the first visit, her sleep schedule had been noted to be highly erratic; coaching on sleep hygiene measures and paying increased attention to her depression seem to have helped. In panel B, red indicates usage <4 hours, green denotes usage ≥4 hours, and black denotes either a large air leak or device malfunction. (*Continued next page.*)

Patterns of Use

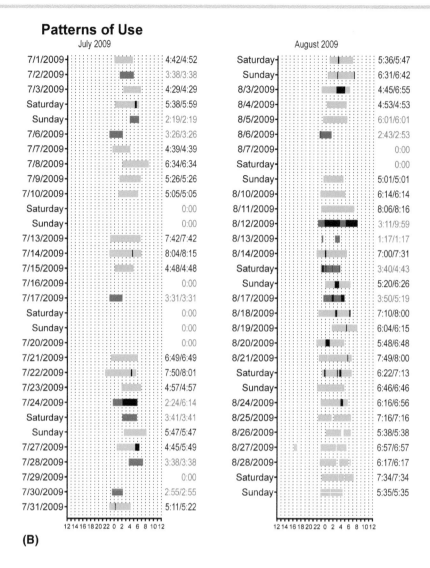

(B)

Figure 28 Continued

APAP Compliance (3/21/2009-9/17/2009)

Device Settings

Therapy Mode: AUTOSET	Minimum Pressure: 5.0 cm H₂O	Maximum Pressure: 20.0 cm H₂O

Pressure (cm H₂O)

Median: 9.6	95th Percentile: 11.4	Maximum: 12.2

Leak (L/min)

Median: 0.0	95th Percentile: 5.4	Maximum: 20.4

AHI and AI (events/hour)

Apnea index: 0.8	AHI: 9.7	% Time in Apnea: 0.3
Hypopnea index: 8.8		

Usage

Used days ≥4 hours: 172	Used days <4 hours: 8	% Used days ≥4 hours: 95
Days not used: 1	Total days: 181	Median daily usage: 6:13
Total hours used: 1,119:51	Average daily usage: 6:11	

(A)

Figure 29 Autotitrating Positive Airway Pressure Compliance Report. (A) This report shows very good treatment compliance, with use on 180 of 181 days and an average daily use of 6 hours and 11 minutes. This autotitrating positive airway pressure (APAP) device has the ability to monitor for apneas, hypopneas, and vibrations in the frequency range of snoring. It calculates an estimated apnea-hypopnea index (AHI), listed here as 9.7. (B) The summary graphs show that the AHI rose over the last 2 months before the follow-up visit on September 17, 2009. It turned out that there was a problem with the function of the mask during those months. Replacement of the mask resulted in an improved AHI, and the patient reported ongoing excellent sleep. AI indicates apnea index.

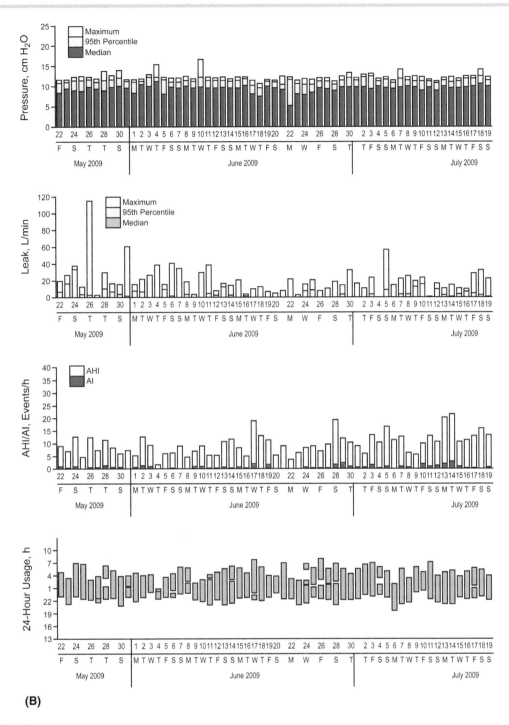

(B)

Figure 29 Continued

either as a stand-alone procedure or in combination with phase 1 procedures (Figure 32).

TREATMENT OF CENTRAL SLEEP APNEA SYNDROME

The primary problem in central sleep apnea syndrome is inadequate or irregular output from the medullary respiratory control center. Treatments involve treating the underlying disease with pharmacologic agents to alter respiratory respon-

siveness, with gases such as oxygen or CO_2 to alter respiratory patterns, or with machines that help regulate ventilation. For example, successful treatment of congestive heart failure reduces the frequency of central apneas. Unfortunately, even in well-compensated congestive heart failure, up to 40% of patients may exhibit CSBP (15). Acetazolamide and even theophylline have been tried to help control central sleep apnea syndrome, but they are rarely successful as long-term treatments (31). Oxygen reliably reduces, but rarely resolves, centrally mediated breathing events. Even when the AHI is

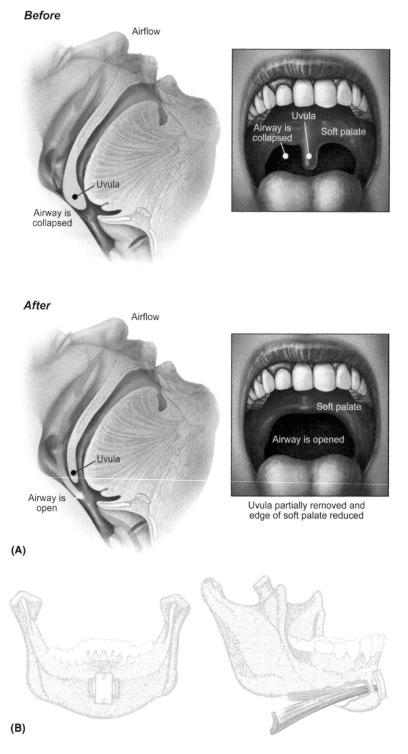

Before

Airflow

Uvula

Airway is collapsed

Uvula

Airway is collapsed

Soft palate

After

Airflow

Uvula

Airway is open

Soft palate

Airway is opened

Uvula partially removed and edge of soft palate reduced

(A)

(B)

Figure 30   Common Surgical Procedures for Obstructive Sleep Apnea Syndrome. (A) The uvulopalatopharyngoplasty opens up the lateral and craniocaudal dimensions of the velopharynx. (Used with permission of Mayo Foundation for Medical Education and Research.) (B) The genioglossus advancement and hyoid myotomy are used to attempt to tighten the retrolingual tissues, increasing the anteroposterior dimension of this area. (Modified from Fairbanks DNF, Fujita S. Snoring and Obstructive Sleep Apnea. New York: Raven Press, 1994. [Used with permission.]) (C) The modified hyoid myotomy and suspension are done to tighten and stabilize the lateral pharyngeal walls. (Modified from Fairbanks DNF, Mickelson SA, Woodson BT. Snoring and Obstructive Sleep Apnea. Philadelphia: Lippincott, Williams & Wilkins, 2003. [Used with permission.]) (D) In maxillomandibular advancement, the entire upper and lower oral cavity and attached soft palatal structures are advanced from the posterior pharyngeal wall, opening the anteroposterior dimension of the airway, and tightening or stabilizing the lateral walls. In patients who begin with a component of retrognathia, this procedure often has a salutary cosmetic effect. (Modified from Fairbanks DNF, Fujita S. Snoring and Obstructive Sleep Apnea. New York: Raven Press, 1994. [Used with permission.])

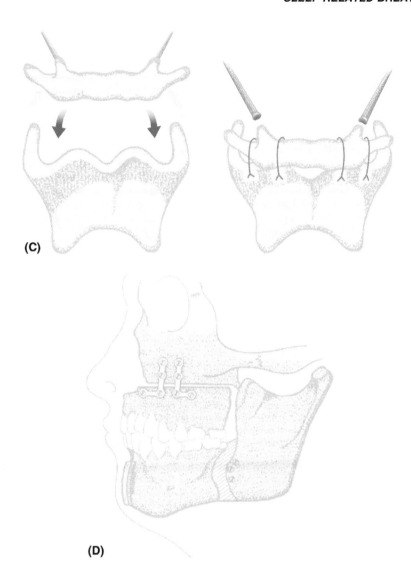

(C)

(D)

Figure 30 Continued

Table 10 Surgical management of obstructive sleep apnea syndrome

Goal of procedure	Obstruction location	Surgical procedure
Bypass all obstructions	NA	Tracheostomy
Modify site of obstruction	Palatal abnormality (tongue normal)	Uvulopalatopharyngoplasty
		Adenotonsillectomy (more often useful in children)
	Palate and base of tongue abnormal	Uvulopalatopharyngoplasty plus genioglossus advancement and hyoid myotomy
		or
		Uvulopalatopharyngoplasty plus temperature-controlled radiofrequency tongue base reduction
	Base of tongue abnormal (palate normal)	Genioglossus advancement and hyoid myotomy
		Temperature-controlled radiofrequency tongue base reduction
	Multiple, especially retrolingual	Maxillomandibular advancement
Indirect surgical treatment	NA	Bariatric surgery

Abbreviation: NA, not applicable.

substantially diminished, arousals and other markers for central sleep apnea persist (11).

Most clinicians have suggested that PAP, either as CPAP, or more recently as adaptive servoventilation, is the first-line therapy. However, a recent randomized controlled trial of CPAP versus best medical therapy did not demonstrate a mortality benefit (32). The results may have been influenced by the fact that in many patients, CPAP did not effectively treat

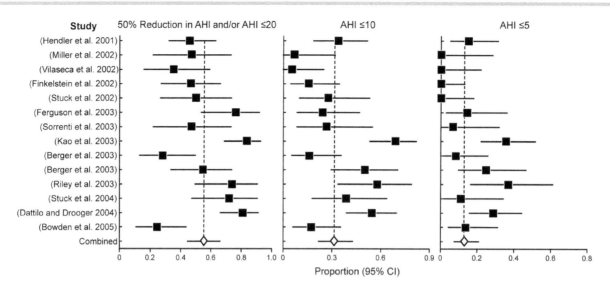

Figure 31 Surgical Cure Rates of Phase 1 Surgical Modifications of the Upper Airway for Obstructive Sleep Apnea. A Forest plot from a meta-analysis of reports of phase 1 surgical procedures (like those shown in Figure 30A-C) shows a relatively low rate of success. When treatment success is defined as a postoperative AHI ≤5 or ≤10, the rates are about 16% and 31%, respectively. These procedures have been performed for more than 30 years, but the selection of ideal candidates remains speculative. Most sleep specialists, because of the disappointing efficacy data, rarely consider these procedures to be the first-line treatment for obstructive sleep apnea. AHI indicates apnea-hypopnea index; CI, confidence interval. [From Elshaug et al [30]. [Used with permission.])

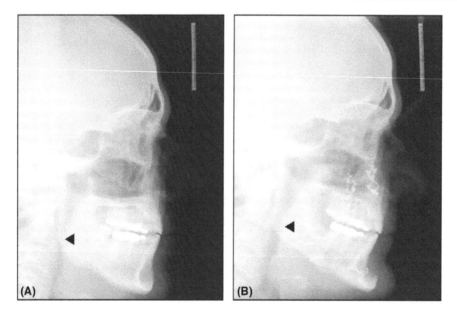

Figure 32 Maxillomandibular Advancement. Typically performed by oral or facial surgeons, maxillomandibular advancement results in a marked increase in the retropharygeal space. (A) Left panel shows a narrowed soft tissue space (arrowhead) in the retrolingual space in this soft tissue lateral film. (B) Right panel shows the increased size of the space after surgery. This patient had a good result, with reduction in the AHI from 46 to 7 and resolution of symptoms.

central sleep apnea, with residual AHI of about 20. In patients in whom CPAP reduced the AHI to <10, there was an improvement in mortality (33). Curiously, even in those patients, the arousal index was not improved, which suggests that the arousals originate from some cyclic input other than respiratory afferents (11,32).

Adaptive servoventilation is more uniformly successful in improving the AHI in patients who have central sleep apnea syndrome (34–37). These devices analyze each breath and adjust the delivered respiratory rate and pressure support in attempts to normalize the breathing pattern (Figure 33). Most studies thus far are small, but adaptive servoventilation

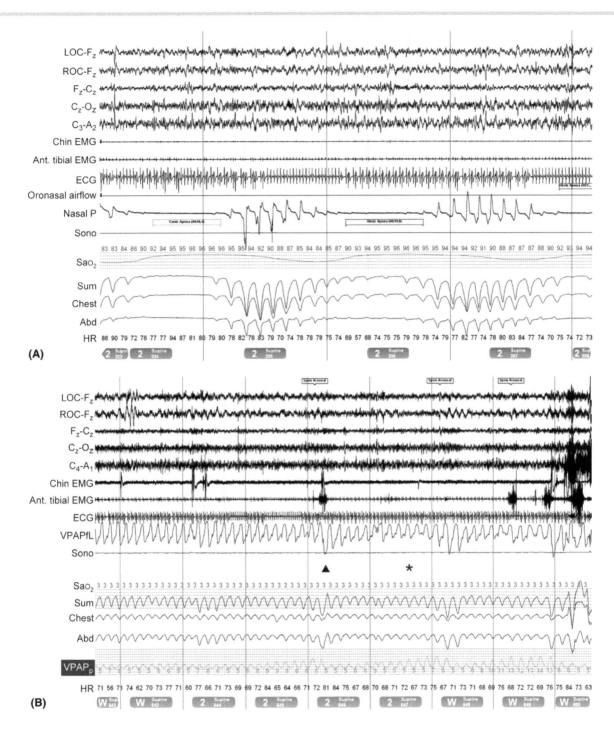

Figure 33 Adaptive Servoventilation in the Treatment of Central and Complex Sleep Apnea Syndromes. (A) The diagnostic polysomnogram of a male patient demonstrates a mix of purely central apneas, obstructive apneas, and hypopneas that often resemble periodic breathing. Application of continuous positive airway pressure (CPAP) eliminated obstructive events, but more than 46 central apneas and central-appearing hypopneas occurred per hour on the best CPAP setting, a situation that has been termed *complex sleep apnea syndrome* (38). (B) This polysomnogram shows the effect of adaptive servoventilation therapy (VPAP AdaptSV; ResMed Corp, Poway, California). The device analyzes each breath and applies an analytic to determine the instantaneous pressure support to apply to try to stabilize the breathing pattern. In the bottom tracing, the end-expiratory pressure is maintained at 5, while the inspiratory positive airway pressure adjusts as seen in the device's pressure channel (VPAPp) in response to the flow recorded in the device pneumotachometer (VPAPfL). Thus, when several breaths with increased tidal volume are seen following an arousal (B, arrowhead), the subsequent pressure support is scaled back until the breathing pattern stabilizes. Later, when there is a decline in tidal volume (B, asterisk [*]), the pressure support increases. With this decline in tidal volume, the inspiratory flow shows a concave pattern and a flattening. This should prompt an increase in the end-expiratory pressure, since it likely indicates flow limitation caused by increased upper airway resistance. End-expiratory pressure stabilizes the upper airway, while the machine selects the appropriate inspiratory pressure and ventilatory rate (Rate) (if need be, in the case of apneas) to try to regulate the breathing pattern. For explanation of labels, see Figure 5.

appears to improve sleep and ejection fraction in heart failure patients; it is also better tolerated than CPAP. Studies are underway to determine whether treatment with adaptive ser-voventilation improves survival in patients with heart failure. Adaptive servoventilation has proven to be an effective way of managing complex sleep apnea syndrome, but there is debate over whether the repetitive central apneas in this variant abate over time while the patient is using CPAP or require adaptive servoventilation for effective treatment (31,39).

REFERENCES

1. Stanchina ML, Ellison K, Malhotra A, et al. The impact of cardiac resynchronization therapy on obstructive sleep apnea in heart failure patients: a pilot study. Chest 2007; 132:433–9. Epub 2007 Jun 15.
2. Kasravi B, Boehmer JP, Leuenberger UA. A noninvasive method for estimating cardiac output using lung to finger circulation time of oxygen. Am J Cardiol 1998; 82:915–7.
3. Iber C, Ancoli-Israel S, Chesson A, Quan SF, editors. The AASM Manual for the Scoring of Sleep and Associated Events: Rules, Terminology and Technical Specifications. Westchester (IL): American Academy of Sleep Medicine, 2007.
4. Younes M. Role of arousals in the pathogenesis of obstructive sleep apnea. Am J Respir Crit Care Med 2004; 169:623–33. Epub 2003 Dec 18.
5. Cui R, Tanigawa T, Sakurai S, Yamagishi K, Iso H. Relationships between sleep-disordered breathing and blood pressure and excessive daytime sleepiness among truck drivers. Hypertens Res 2006; 29:605–10.
6. Wilson K, Stoohs RA, Mulrooney TF, et al. The snoring spectrum: acoustic assessment of snoring sound intensity in 1,139 individuals undergoing polysomnography. Chest 1999; 115:762–70.
7. Sin DD, Fitzgerald F, Parker JD, Newton G, Floras JS, Bradley TD. Risk factors for central and obstructive sleep apnea in 450 men and women with congestive heart failure. Am J Respir Crit Care Med 1999; 160:1101–6.
8. Roehrs T, Zorick F, Wittig R, Conway W, Roth T. Predictors of objective level of daytime sleepiness in patients with sleep-related breathing disorders. Chest 1989; 95:1202–6.
9. Walker JM, Farney RJ, Rhondeau SM, et al. Chronic opioid use is a risk factor for the development of central sleep apnea and ataxic breathing. J Clin Sleep Med 2007; 3:455–61. Erratum in: J Clin Sleep Med 2007; 3.
10. Lee P, Su YN, Yu CJ, Yang PC, Wu HD. *PHOX2B* mutation-confirmed congenital central hypoventilation syndrome in a Chinese family: presentation from newborn to adulthood. Chest 2009; 135:537–44.
11. Ruttanaumpawan P, Logan AG, Floras JS, Bradley TD; CANPAP Investigators. Effect of continuous positive airway pressure on sleep structure in heart failure patients with central sleep apnea. Sleep 2009; 32:91–8.
12. Schellenberg JB, Maislin G, Schwab RJ. Physical findings and the risk for obstructive sleep apnea: the importance of oropharyngeal structures. Am J Respir Crit Care Med 2000; 162(2 Pt 1):740–8.
13. Friedman M, Soans R, Gurpinar B, Lin HC, Joseph NJ. Interexaminer agreement of Friedman tongue positions for staging of obstructive sleep apnea/hypopnea syndrome. Otolaryngol Head Neck Surg 2008; 139:372–7.
14. Javaheri S, Parker TJ, Wexler L, et al. Occult sleep-disordered breathing in stable congestive heart failure. Ann Intern Med 1995; 122:487–92. Erratum in: Ann Intern Med 1995; 123:77.
15. Javaheri S. Central sleep apnea in congestive heart failure: prevalence, mechanisms, impact, and therapeutic options. Semin Respir Crit Care Med 2005; 26:44–55.
16. Brack T, Thuer I, Clarenbach CF, et al. Daytime Cheyne-Stokes respiration in ambulatory patients with severe congestive heart failure is associated with increased mortality. Chest 2007; 132:1463–71. Epub 2007 Jul 23.
17. Bassetti C, Aldrich MS. Sleep apnea in acute cerebrovascular diseases: final report on 128 patients. Sleep 1999; 22:217–23.
18. Morgenthaler TI. The quest for stability in an unstable world: adaptive servoventilation in opioid induced complex sleep apnea syndrome. J Clin Sleep Med 2008; 4:321–3.
19. Teichtahl H, Wang D. Sleep-disordered breathing with chronic opioid use. Expert Opin Drug Saf 2007; 6:641–9.
20. Farney RJ, Walker JM, Cloward TV, Rhondeau S. Sleep-disordered breathing associated with long-term opioid therapy. Chest 2003; 123:632–9.
21. Grigg-Damberger M, Wells A. Central congenital hypoventilation syndrome: changing face of a less mysterious but more complex genetic disorder. Semin Respir Crit Care Med 2009; 30:262–74. Epub 2009 May 18.
22. AASM. The International Classification of Sleep Disorders: Diagnostic and Coding Manual. 2nd ed. Westchester, IL: American Academy of Sleep Medicine, 2005.
23. Sampol G, Munoz X, Sagales MT, et al. Long-term efficacy of dietary weight loss in sleep apnoea/hypopnoea syndrome. Eur Respir J 1998; 12:1156–9.
24. Wenzel S, Smith E, Leiacker R, Fischer Y. [Efficacy and longterm compliance of the vest preventing the supine position in patients with obstructive sleep apnea]. Laryngorhinootologie 2007; 86: 579–83. German.
25. Ferguson K. Oral appliance therapy for obstructive sleep apnea: finally evidence you can sink your teeth into. Am J Respir Crit Care Med 2001; 163:1294–5.
26. Morgenthaler TI, Kapen S, Lee-Chiong T, et al; Standards of Practice Committee; American Academy of Sleep Medicine. Practice parameters for the medical therapy of obstructive sleep apnea. Sleep 2006; 29:1031–5.
27. Kushida CA, Morgenthaler TI, Littner MR, et al; American Academy of Sleep. Practice parameters for the treatment of snoring and obstructive sleep apnea with oral appliances: an update for 2005. Sleep 2006; 29:240–3.
28. Kushida CA, Chediak A, Berry RB, et al; Positive Airway Pressure Titration Task Force; American Academy of Sleep Medicine. Clinical guidelines for the manual titration of positive airway pressure in patients with obstructive sleep apnea. J Clin Sleep Med 2008; 4:157–71.
29. Weaver TE, Chasens ER. Continuous positive airway pressure treatment for sleep apnea in older adults. Sleep Med Rev 2007; 11:99–111. Epub 2007 Feb 1.
30. Elshaug AG, Moss JR, Southcott AM, Hiller JE. Redefining success in airway surgery for obstructive sleep apnea: a meta analysis and synthesis of the evidence. Sleep 2007; 30:461–7.
31. Allam JS, Morgenthaler TI. Central sleep apnea syndrome. BMJ Point of Care 5 June 2008.
32. Bradley TD, Logan AG, Kimoff RJ, et al; CANPAP Investigators. Continuous positive airway pressure for central sleep apnea and heart failure. N Engl J Med 2005; 353:2025–33.
33. Arzt M, Floras JS, Logan AG, et al; CANPAP Investigators. Suppression of central sleep apnea by continuous positive airway pressure and transplant-free survival in heart failure: a post hoc analysis of the Canadian Continuous Positive Airway Pressure for Patients with Central Sleep Apnea and Heart Failure Trial (CANPAP). Circulation 2007; 115:3173–80. Epub 2007 Jun 11.
34. Oldenburg O, Schmidt A, Lamp B, et al. Adaptive servoventilation improves cardiac function in patients with chronic heart failure and Cheyne-Stokes respiration. Eur J Heart Fail 2008; 10:581–6. Epub 2008 May 16.
35. Allam JS, Olson EJ, Gay PC, Morgenthaler TI. Efficacy of adaptive servoventilation in treatment of complex and central sleep apnea syndromes. Chest 2007; 132:1839–46.
36. Philippe C, Stoica-Herman M, Drouot X, et al. Compliance with and effectiveness of adaptive servoventilation versus continuous

positive airway pressure in the treatment of Cheyne-Stokes respiration in heart failure over a six month period. Heart 2006; 92: 337–42. Epub 2005 Jun 17.

37. Pepperell JC, Maskell NA, Jones DR, et al. A randomized controlled trial of adaptive ventilation for Cheyne-Stokes breathing in heart failure. Am J Respir Crit Care Med 2003; 168:1109–14. Epub 2003 Aug 19.

38. Morgenthaler TI, Kagramanov V, Hanak V, Decker PA. Complex sleep apnea syndrome: is it a unique clinical syndrome? Sleep 2006; 29:1203–9.

39. Morgenthaler TI, Gay PC, Gordon N, Brown LK. Adaptive servo-ventilation versus noninvasive positive pressure ventilation for central, mixed, and complex sleep apnea syndromes. Sleep 2007; 30:468–75.

7

Narcolepsy

Michael H. Silber, MBChB, FCP (SA)

ABBREVIATIONS

CSF, cerebrospinal fluid

hcrt, hypocretin

HLA, human leukocyte antigen

REM, rapid eye movement

Narcolepsy has been recognized as a distinct condition for 130 years. First described by the German neuropsychiatrist Karl Friedrich Otto Westphal and the French physician Jean Baptiste Gélineau, narcolepsy is the classic example of a disorder of excessive sleep (1). It also illustrates how advances in the knowledge of sleep physiology have led to dramatic insights into the pathogenesis of a sleep disorder. Parallel with the understanding of the mechanisms of the disease has come the development of new medications for its treatment.

The prevalence of narcolepsy in various American and European studies ranges from 26 to 67 per 100,000 population (2), indicating that one might expect to find about 400 persons with narcolepsy in an area with a population of 1 million at any one time. The incidence rate of narcolepsy has been calculated as 1.4 per 100,000 population per year, which translates to the diagnosis of 14 new patients each year in a population of 1 million (3). The disorder most frequently commences between the ages of 10 and 20 years, and rarely starts after age 40 (Figure 1). It is slightly more common in men than in women (1.5:1) (3).

CLINICAL FEATURES

The essential clinical characteristic of narcolepsy is excessive sleepiness. Although this symptom is not specific for the disorder, the sleepiness inherent to narcolepsy is usually more severe than that in many other conditions causing hypersomnia. Persons with narcolepsy can fall asleep in any sedentary situation, such as while reading, studying, watching television, or sitting in an audience. Driving can be especially problematic because persons with narcolepsy may fall asleep while stopped at red traffic lights and frequently experience near-accidents. Automatic behavior may occur during drowsiness, such as continuing to type or write but producing only meaningless strings of letters.

The most specific symptom of narcolepsy is cataplexy, which consists of sudden, transient, bilateral muscle weakness precipitated by emotion. In a full attack of cataplexy, all the skeletal muscles are paralyzed with the exception of the extraocular muscles and the diaphragm. Despite an inability to speak, the patient remains fully conscious and perceives normal sensation. More common are partial cataplectic attacks

with a sudden buckling of the knees or with sagging of the face, jaw, or neck that may be accompanied by slurred speech. Attacks usually last from seconds to minutes. Neurological examination during a cataplectic event reveals transient loss of deep tendon reflexes. The most common precipitant emotion is laughter, related either to the patient hearing or telling a joke (Figure 2) (4). Less commonly, cataplexy can be induced by other emotions, such as surprise, anger, or excitement, which sometimes occur during a sporting event or a recreational activity such as fishing or hunting. Depending on the definition of the symptom and the population being studied, cataplexy has been found to occur in 64% to 80% of patients with narcolepsy (3,5). It usually commences after the onset of sleepiness, most often within 4 years but sometimes as much as 10 or more years after disease onset (Figure 3) (6). In some patients, the frequency of cataplectic attacks appears to decrease with age, but this decline may occur as those patients learn how to control precipitant emotions. In other patients the attacks seem to occur more frequently with age and may be less clearly precipitated by emotion.

Sleepiness, cataplexy, hypnagogic hallucinations, and sleep paralysis have long been considered the tetrad of symptoms of narcolepsy. However, hypnagogic hallucinations and sleep paralysis are neither specific nor particularly sensitive for the diagnosis, and thus they should be considered ancillary clinical features with low diagnostic usefulness. Hypnagogic hallucinations, experienced in the transition between wakefulness and sleep, are usually visual but may be auditory, tactile, or vestibular. Similar experiences at sleep termination are known as hypnopompic hallucinations. Sleep paralysis refers to the transient inability to move, with preserved consciousness, at sleep onset or on wakening. Attacks of sleep paralysis may be accompanied by hallucinations and can often be aborted by touching the patient. About 25% of the normal population report having had hallucinations at sleep onset, and 7% describe episodes of sleep paralysis (7,8). In contrast, about 60% of patients with narcolepsy and cataplexy experience hypnagogic hallucinations and 66% experience sleep paralysis. However, only 32% of patients who have narcolepsy without cataplexy report having hypnagogic hallucinations and only 7% report sleep paralysis (9).

Paradoxically, patients with narcolepsy frequently complain of poor-quality sleep at night. Sleep is fragmented with frequent awakenings, periodic limb movements are common, and dream enactment behavior may occur. Rapid eye movement (REM) sleep occurs earlier than normal and is often fragmented with multiple periods of REM sleep evenly distributed throughout the night (Figure 4). The body mass index

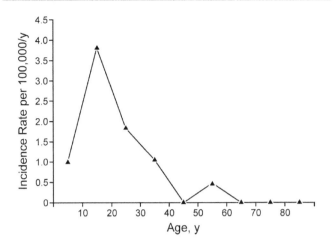

Figure 1 Age of Onset of Narcolepsy. The incidence rate of narcolepsy varies by age, as illustrated by this graph of results from a population-based study. Narcolepsy generally commences in childhood or young adulthood, with the highest rate occurring between the ages of 10 and 20 years. The highest rates after that occur in persons younger than 10 years of age or between 20 and 30 years of age. Onset of idiopathic narcolepsy after age 40 is rare. (Adapted from Silber et al. [3]. [Used with permission.])

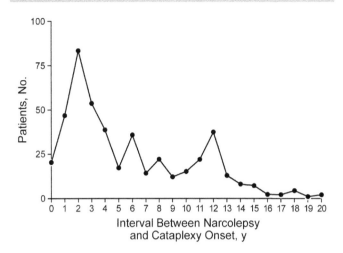

Figure 3 Onset of Cataplexy in Relation to Onset of Sleepiness in Patients With Narcolepsy. After the onset of sleepiness in patients with narcolepsy, there is usually a gap of a year or longer before the onset of cataplexy. Cataplexy commences simultaneous to or within a few years after the development of sleepiness in most patients. However, in a few patients cataplexy first develops one or more decades after the start of narcolepsy. (Adapted from Okun ML et al. [6]. [Used with permission.])

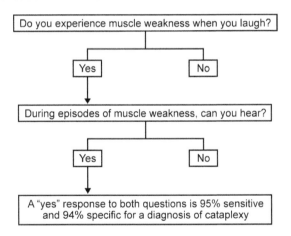

Figure 2 Algorithm for Diagnosis of Cataplexy. Because many normal persons endorse feelings of weakness with intense laughter, the clinical diagnosis of cataplexy can sometimes be challenging. This simple algorithm, based on a study of 78 patients and 78 control subjects, is highly sensitive and specific for the diagnosis. (Data from Moore WR et al. [4].)

identified, many with pathology in the hypothalamus or in the region of the third ventricle. Deeper understanding of the pathophysiology of the disorder has occurred in three phases, starting in 1960.

REM Sleep Abnormalities

Seven years after the discovery of REM sleep in 1953, researchers noted that it occurred earlier than expected in the sleep of patients with narcolepsy (11). The normal mean REM latency (time from sleep onset to the first period of REM sleep) is about 90 minutes, but REM latency is considerably shortened in patients with narcolepsy. This phenomenon is made use of in the multiple sleep latency test, in which the presence of REM sleep during daytime naps is used as a test for narcolepsy. In addition to having abnormal timing of REM sleep, persons with narcolepsy have a dissociation of REM phenomena, with cataplexy representing the muscle paralysis of REM sleep intruding into wakefulness and hypnagogic hallucinations representing the dreams of REM sleep occurring atypically at wake-sleep transition. Abnormally increased muscle activity may also be present during REM sleep.

Association With the HLA System

A 1984 report that Japanese patients with narcolepsy were highly likely to carry the human leukocyte antigen (HLA) haplotype DR2 initiated a different direction of research (12). This initial finding was later confirmed in white patients with narcolepsy, but less consistently in African Americans with the disorder. On the basis of these data, genetic studies revealed that the actual linkage was to the DQ1 antigen, specifically the DQB1*0602 subtype (Figure 5) (13). Of persons with narcolepsy who are affected with clear-cut cataplexy, 85% to 93% test positive for HLA DQB1*0602, compared with 35% to 56% of

of patients with narcolepsy is higher than that of controls, and patients often report a sudden increase in weight around the time of onset of the disorder (10).

PATHOPHYSIOLOGY

During the first 80 years after narcolepsy was initially recognized, its clinical features were fully described. Rare cases of narcolepsy associated with other neurological disorders were

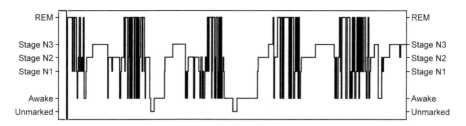

Figure 4 Graphical Representation of Nocturnal Sleep in Narcolepsy. The nocturnal sleep of a patient with narcolepsy is typically unsustained, with frequent awakenings. The first rapid eye movement (REM) sleep period may occur earlier than expected. Rapid eye movement sleep may be fragmented, with REM sleep periods evenly distributed throughout the night rather than clustering in the second half. (Adapted from Krahn LE, Black JL, Silber MH. Narcolepsy: new understanding of irresistible sleep. Mayo Clin Proc 2001 76: 185–94. [Used with permission.])

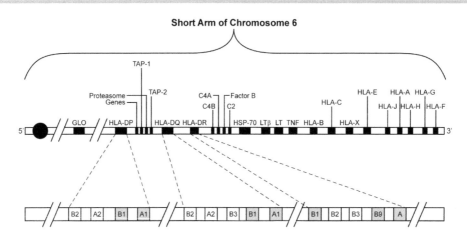

Figure 5 Structure of the Short Arm of Chromosome 6. This figure illustrates the location of the major histocompatability complex in humans at the HLA locus on the short arm of chromosome 6. Approximately 90% of patients with cataplexy secondary to narcolepsy carry the HLA DQB1*0602 allele compared with about 20% of controls. This relationship strongly supports the hypothesis that the disorder is of autoimmune origin. (From Cruse JM, Lewis RE. Illustrated Dictionary of Immunology. 3rd ed. Boca Raton: CRC Press, 2009. [Used with permission.])

those without cataplexy and about 20% of the white control population. Despite this close relationship to a genetically determined biological marker, environmental factors are believed to play a more important role in the pathogenesis of narcolepsy. Only 1% to 2% of first-degree relatives of narcoleptic patients will also have the disease, whereas 70% to 75% of monozygotic twins are discordant for the disorder (14). Diseases associated with a specific HLA subtype are almost always autoimmune in nature, but searches for general serum autoimmune markers in narcolepsy have been negative (15) and there are no reported conventional changes identified by magnetic resonance imaging or cerebrospinal fluid (CSF) analysis that suggest narcolepsy is an inflammatory disease of the brain. No antibodies to any component of the hypocretin (hcrt) system (see below) have been detected in the serum or CSF of persons with narcolepsy (16). Several other studies have provided some supportive evidence for the autoimmune hypothesis of narcolepsy. Purified serum immunoglobulin G from patients resulted in increased contractile response of mouse bladder detrusor muscle to cholinergic stimulation compared

with immunoglobulin G from controls (17). In another study, CSF immunoglobulin G from patients that was incubated with homogenized rat hypothalamic protein extract demonstrated significant binding compared with that of controls (18). A recent study linked narcolepsy to a specific polymorphism of the T-cell receptor α locus, part of the protein-binding HLA molecules (19). Streptococcal antibodies were found at higher titers in the serum of patients with narcolepsy commencing less than 3 years before testing compared to patients with a longer duration of disease and normal control subjects (20). Despite these tantalizing hints, no definitive proof has been found to confirm an autoimmune mechanism for the pathogenesis of narcolepsy.

Association With the Hypocretin (orexin) System

The next phase in understanding narcolepsy emerged from the painstaking work of Emmanuel Mignot and his team at Stanford University, who were interested in determining the cause of autosomal recessive narcolepsy in dogs (Figure 6). In 1999

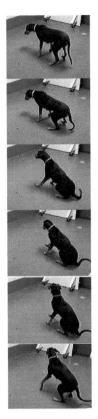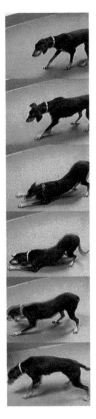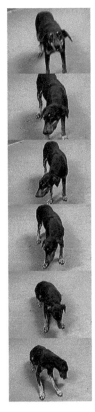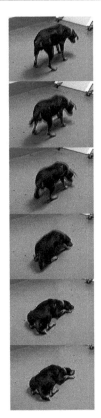

Figure 6 Cataplexy in Narcoleptic Dogs. This series of consecutive photographs shows a narcoleptic Doberman pinscher undergoing food-elicited cataplexy tests at the Center for Narcolepsy in the Stanford School of Medicine at Stanford University. The emotional stimuli of the sight and smell of pellets of food induce cataplexy in the dog, which is awake but unable to move. Unlike narcolepsy in humans, narcolepsy in dogs is generally inherited as an autosomal recessive trait due to the genetic absence of the hypocretin-2 receptor. (From Nishino S. Clinical and neurobiological aspects of narcolepsy. Sleep Med 2007; 8: 373-99. [Used with permission.])

they discovered that the disorder was caused by a deletion in the hcrt (orexin) receptor-2 gene (21). Hypocretins, first discovered in 1998, are peptide neurotransmitters secreted by the posterolateral hypothalamus (Figure 7). About the same time, another group of investigators, working with an hcrt knockout mouse model, serendipitously recognized that episodes of either REM sleep or cataplexy developed in the mutant mice while they were awake (22). In humans, hcrt-1 (orexin-A) concentrations in the CSF can be measured. In patients with narcolepsy and associated cataplexy, 87% have undetectable hcrt-1 levels in the CSF compared with 14% of patients who have narcolepsy without cataplexy and 2% of neurological controls (Figure 8) (23). Human autopsy studies have documented the loss of >90% of the hcrt-secreting cells in the hypothalamus with evidence of gliosis (Figure 9) (24). The mechanism of this cell loss remains undetermined. These findings presumably explain rare reports of secondary narcolepsy arising from lesions of the hypothalamus or pituitary gland (Figure 10) (25).

DIAGNOSIS

The presence of excessive sleepiness and definite cataplexy precipitated by laughter is highly suggestive of a diagnosis of narcolepsy. However, in view of the lifelong nature of the disorder and the need for treatment with often potentially addictive medication, objective confirmation of the disorder is advisable. If cataplexy is not present, further testing is essential. When transient loss of deep tendon reflexes can be

Preprohypocretin Polypeptides

MNLPSTKVSWAAVTLLLLLLLLLPPALLSSGAAAQPL
PDCCRQKTCSCRLYELLHGAGNHAAGILTLGKRR
SGPPGLQGRLQRLLQASGNHAAGILTMGRRAGAE
PAPRPCLGRRCSAPAAASVAPGGQSGI

Black letters = N-terminus peptide
Red letters = Hypocretin 1
Tan letters = Linker between hypocretin 1 and 2
Green letters = Hypocretin 2
Blue letters = C-terminus (test peptide 1)
Pink letters = C-terminus (test peptide 2)
Bold letters (Blue and Pink) = C-terminus (test peptide 3)
<u>Underlined</u> letters = C-terminus (test peptide 4)

Figure 7 The Structure of Preprohypocretin. This figure represents the amino acid structures of preprohypocretin and the two active neurotransmitters, hypocretin 1 and 2. Serum and cerebrospinal fluid of patients with narcolepsy have been tested unsuccessfully for antibodies to each component of the molecule indicated on the figure. Antibodies to hypocretin receptor 1 and 2 were also not detected. Further work to confirm or refute the autoimmune hypothesis of narcolepsy should concentrate on cellular immune mechanisms and other components of the hypocretin-synthesizing neurons. (From Silber MH, Black JL, Krahn LE, Fredrickson PA. Autoimmune Studies in Narcolepsy. In: Bassetti CL, Billiard M, Mignot E. Narcolepsy and Hypersomnia. New York [NY]: Informa Healthcare, 2007. [Used with permission.])

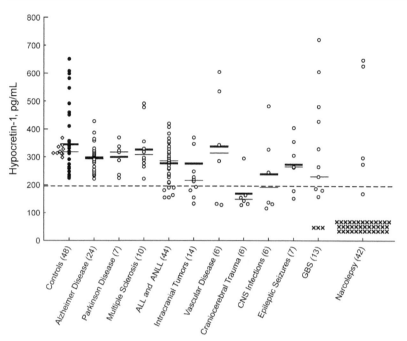

Figure 8 Hypocretin Levels in Patients With Narcolepsy vs in Controls. This graph indicates hypocretin-1 levels in the cerebrospinal fluid of 42 patients who had narcolepsy with cataplexy, 137 patients with a variety of other neurological disorders, and 48 normal controls. As can be seen, 88% (37/42) of narcoleptic patients had levels <110 pg/mL. The only control patients with such low levels were a small subset of the patients with Guillain-Barré syndrome. Some patients with a variety of other neurological disorders had levels between the lower limit of normal (190 pg/mL) and 110 pg/mL. It should be noted that other studies have demonstrated that fewer than 20% of patients who have narcolepsy without cataplexy have low hypocretin-1 levels. ALL indicates acute lymphoblastic leukemia; ANLL, acute nonlymphoblastic leukemia; CNS, central nervous system; GBS, Guillain-Barré syndrome. (From Ripley B et al. [23]. Used with permission.])

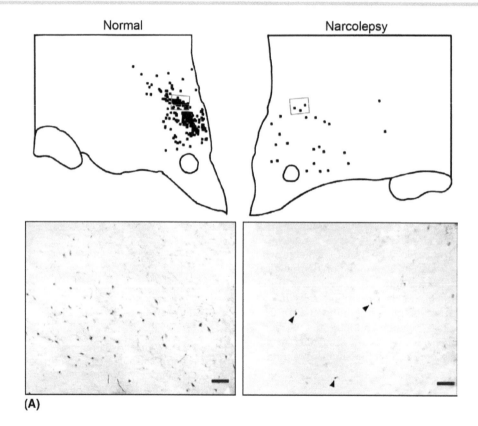

(A)

Figure 9 Loss of Hypothalamic Hypocretin-Synthesizing Cells With Gliosis in Narcolepsy. The autopsy study described here was based on four narcoleptic and 12 control brains. Figure 9A shows the number of neurons in the perifornical and dorsomedial hypothalamus immunolabeled for hypocretin in a patient with narcolepsy (right) and in a control subject (left). The lower panels show low-power photomicrographs of outlined areas in the top images. Note the marked loss (average, 93%) of neurons (arrowheads [right image]) in the narcoleptic patient. Figure 9B shows the same region demonstrating astrocytes stained for glial fibrillary acidic protein (GFAP). Note the increased number of GFAP-labeled astrocytes in the narcoleptic patient (right), indicating the presence of gliosis, which suggests acquired loss of neurons in the region. (From Thannickal TC et al. [24]. [Used with permission.])

Normal | Narcolepsy

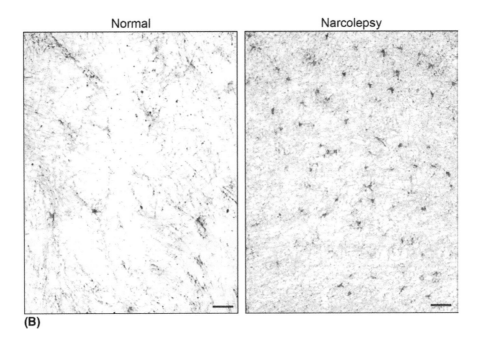

(B)

Figure 9 Continued

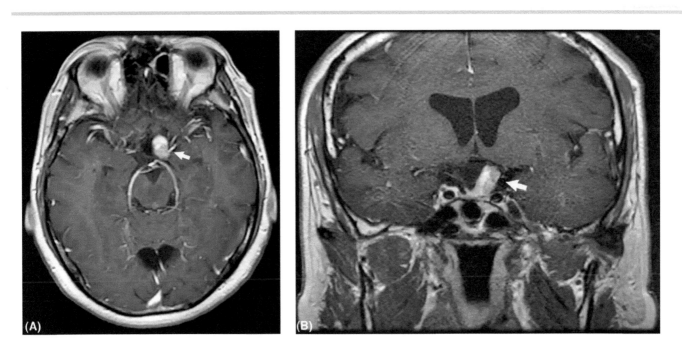

(A) (B)

Figure 10 Suprasellar Pituitary Tumor Causing Narcolepsy. (A and B) These magnetic resonance imaging scans are of a patient in whom sleepiness without cataplexy developed at the age of 17 years. Headaches and visual loss led to the diagnosis of a suprasellar pituitary adenoma (A and B [arrow]) at the age of 23 years. He underwent transsphenoidal partial resection of the tumor, followed by radiation therapy. A multiple sleep latency test showed a mean sleep latency of 2.6 minutes with REM (rapid eye movement) sleep occurring within 15 minutes of sleep onset on all four naps. Narcolepsy was diagnosed. The magnetic resonance imaging scans are those of T1-weighted images in the axial and coronal planes with gadolinium enhancement. They show a residual left-sided sellar and suprasellar mass. Secondary narcolepsy is uncommon but usually associated with hypothalamic or pituitary pathology and presumably results from destruction of hypocretin-synthesizing cells or the interruption of hypocretin outflow tracts.

demonstrated during a presumed cataplectic attack, the diagnosis can be firmly established. For most patients, a multiple sleep latency test should be performed (see chapter 5) (Figure 11). The presence of two or more sleep-onset REM periods is highly suggestive of narcolepsy, as long as the test has been performed under standardized conditions, excluding the confounding effects of sleep deprivation, sudden withdrawal of REM suppressant medication, or obstructive sleep apnea (Figure 12). The mean sleep latency should be less than eight minutes and is usually less than five (26). Alternatively, the diagnosis can be

Multiple Sleep Latency Test

Nap Time	Initial Sleep Latency, min[a]	Unequivocal Sleep Latency, min[b]	REM Latency, min	Total Sleep, min
9:02	2.5	2.5	2.5	15.0
11:02	2.0	2.0	2.0	14.5
13:06	3.0	3.0	3.0	15.5
14:58	2.5	2.5	2.5	15.0
Mean	2.5	2.5		

[a]First epoch scored with any sleep stage.
[b]First epoch contiguous with >75 seconds of any sleep stage plus sleep spindles, K complexes, or REM (rapid eye movement) sleep.

Summary:
A multiple sleep latency test was performed after overnight polysommography that revealed an adequate total sleep time of 475 minutes and a normal apnea-hypopnea index of 2 per hour. The urine drug screen was negative. The mean sleep latency was 2.5 minutes. Sleep-onset REM sleep was observed in all 4 nap opportunities.

Clinical Interpretation:
The study shows the presence of severe, excessive daytime sleepiness. These findings are diagnostic of narcolepsy.

Figure 11   Multiple Sleep Latency Report in a Patient With Narcolepsy. This report of a multiple sleep latency test of a 25-year-old man shows the typical findings associated with severe narcolepsy. The neurophysiological marker of narcolepsy is REM (rapid eye movement) sleep occurring within 15 minutes of sleep onset. It is measured by the multiple sleep latency test, in which patients are given 4 or 5 nap opportunities every 2 hours over the course of a day under standardized conditions. A patient who falls asleep within 20 minutes after the lights are turned off is allowed 15 minutes of sleep to assess for the presence of REM sleep. REM sleep recorded on 2 or more naps within 15 minutes of sleep onset is diagnostic for narcolepsy as long as the test has been adequately performed, with the exclusion of confounders such as severe obstructive sleep apnea, withdrawal of REM-suppressant drugs, or sleep deprivation. In addition, the mean sleep latency over the 4 naps is calculated; more than 90% of patients with narcolepsy have a mean latency of less than 8 minutes, with most having less than 5 minutes.

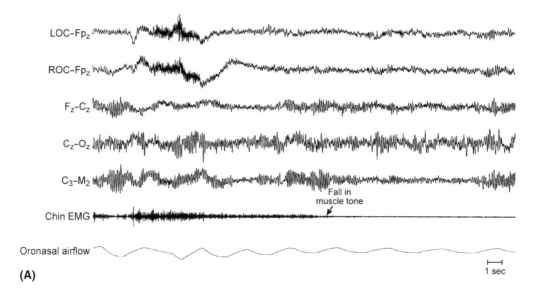

(A)

Figure 12   REM-Onset Polysomnogram. (A-C) These three consecutive 30-second epochs from a multiple sleep latency test illustrate a sleep-onset rapid eye movement (REM) period in a patient with narcolepsy. The patient rapidly transitions from wakefulness to REM sleep one minute after lights have been turned off. EMG indicates electromyogram; LOC, left outer canthus; ROC, right outer canthus.

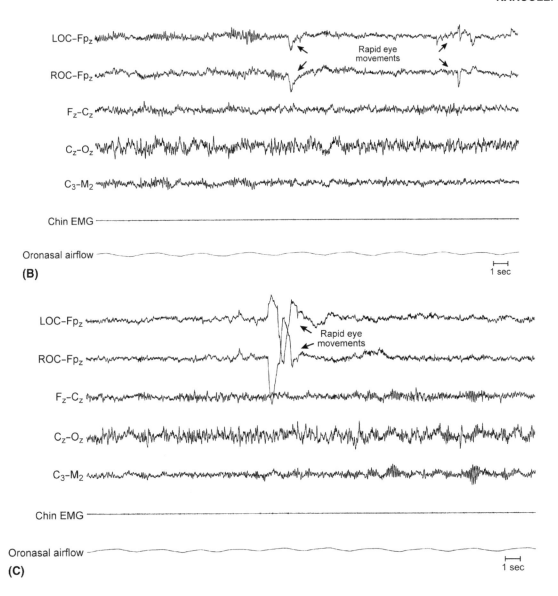

Figure 12 Continued

confirmed by demonstrating absent hcrt-1 in the CSF, but this test is currently available only as a research tool. It is also of note that the sensitivity of a positive result in the absence of cataplexy is very low.

The broad differential diagnosis of narcolepsy encompasses most other causes of excessive sleepiness (Table 1 and Figure 13). In particular, one must rule out obstructive sleep apnea, insufficient sleep syndrome, and the sedating effects of medications, such as opioids, benzodiazepines, and dopaminergic agents. The disorder most similar to narcolepsy and most likely to be confused with it is idiopathic hypersomnia. This condition is characterized by an absence of cataplexy, the exclusion of other causes of somnolence, and multiple sleep latency test results that show a short mean sleep latency but fewer than two sleep-onset REM periods. Idiopathic hypersomnia is currently divided into two subcategories: idiopathic hypersomnia with long sleep time and idiopathic hypersomnia

Table 1   Causes of excessive daytime sleepiness

Extrinsic causes
   Sleep deprivation (insufficient sleep syndrome)
   Drug-related hypersomnia
   Shift work disorder
   Jet lag disorder
   Environmental sleep disorder

Intrinsic causes
   Sleep-related breathing disorder
   Narcolepsy
   Idiopathic hypersomnia
   Restless legs syndrome and periodic limb movement disorder
   Circadian rhythm sleep disorders (including delayed sleep phase disorder)
   Recurrent hypersomnia (including Kleine-Levin syndrome)

From Silber MH, Krahn LE, Morgenthaler TI. Sleep Medicine in Clinical Practice. New York: Taylor & Francis, 2004. (Used with permission of Mayo Foundation for Medical Education and Research.)

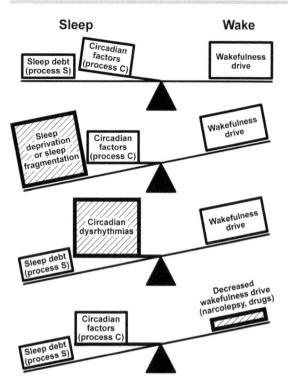

Figure 13 Mechanisms of Sleepiness. The balance between sleep and wakefulness is maintained through factors that promote alertness and factors that induce sleep. The wakefulness drive depends primarily on the release of the neurotransmitter hypocretin (orexin), which in turn activates bioamines in the brainstem. Narcolepsy is the classic example of a disorder of excessive sleep caused by hypocretin deficiency. Medications affecting monoamines, such as histamine-1 receptor antagonists, can also induce sleep. The sleep drive depends on circadian (process C) and homeostatic (process S) factors. Circadian dysrhythmias, such as delayed sleep phase disorder or shift work sleep disorder, can cause sleepiness. Sleepiness can also be caused by increased homeostatic sleep drive (sleep debt) from sleep deprivation or sleep fragmentation caused, for example, by obstructive sleep apnea. (From Silber MH, Krahn LE, Morgenthaler TI. Sleep Medicine in Clinical Practice. New York: Taylor & Francis, 2004. [Used with permission of Mayo Foundation for Medical Education and Research.])

without long sleep time (26). In the former condition, nocturnal sleep is deep and undisturbed, lasting at least 10 hours. Waking in the morning is difficult and may be accompanied by transient confusion referred to as sleep drunkenness. Patients take long but unrefreshing naps. Idiopathic hypersomnia without long sleep time has none of these associated features. More recent work has cast doubt on the validity of subdividing the condition in this manner (27).

MANAGEMENT

Until recently, sympathomimetic agents were the mainstay of treatment for narcolepsy. First introduced in the 1930s, these medications enhance the release of monoamines into the synaptic cleft and block their reuptake. Methylphenidate has been used the most frequently, but various amphetamine preparations have proved useful in more severely affected patients (Table 2). Although these drugs are clearly effective in most

Table 2 Commonly used short-acting and long-acting stimulants

Medication	Typical daily starting dose	Recommended maximum daily dose
Short-acting stimulants		
Methylphenidate	30 mg	100 mg[a]
Dextroamphetamine	15 mg	100 mg[a]
Mixed dextroamphetamine and levoamphetamine (Adderall)	20 mg	60 mg[b]
Methamphetamine	15 mg	80 mg[a]
Long-acting stimulants		
Extended-release methylphenidate	20 mg	60 mg[b]
Extended-release methylphenidate (Concerta)	18 mg	72 mg (for attention-deficit/hyperactivity disorder)[b]
Extended-release dextroamphetamine (Dexedrine Spansule)		60 mg[b]
Extended-release mixed dextroamphetamine and levoamphetamine (Adderall XR)	20 mg	60 mg[c]
Modafinil	100 mg	400 mg[b]

[a] American Academy of Sleep Medicine recommendations (28). (Note that some of these maximum doses exceed the manufacturer's recommendations.)
[b] Manufacturer's recommendations.
[c] Derived from recommended maximum dose of short-acting Adderall.
From Silber MH, Krahn LE, Morgenthaler TI. Sleep Medicine in Clinical Practice. New York: Taylor & Francis, 2004. (Used with permission of Mayo Foundation for Medical Education and Research.)

patients, adverse effects often limit their use. With doses high enough to relieve sleepiness, patients may experience undesirable sympathetic side effects, including irritability, tremor, palpitations, anorexia, and weight loss. Amphetamines, especially in high doses, may lead to the development of psychosis in an occasional patient (29). Amphetamine preparations have been associated with sudden death in children, and they should not be used in patients with long QT syndrome or cardiomyopathy. Short-acting agents may result in severe peak and trough effects, with the patient experiencing rapid transitions between unpleasantly enhanced alertness and severe sleepiness (Figure 14). These effects can be attenuated by substituting slow-release preparations, which are available for both methylphenidate and the amphetamines. These medications are potentially dependence-producing and tolerance may occur.

The development of the novel central nervous system stimulant modafinil has led to a different approach to the management of narcolepsy (Figure 15) (30,31). The mechanism of action of modafinil has not been firmly established, but it is now the most commonly prescribed first-line agent for treatment of narcolepsy. It is taken once or twice daily and does not have the peak and trough effects of conventional stimulants. Despite occasional headaches, nausea, and rhinitis, it is relatively free of side effects. Modafinil is probably not addictive. However, it is a milder stimulant than the sympathomimetic agents, so patients with moderately severe narcolepsy often find that it provides inadequate alertness. Modafinil is metabolized through the cytochrome P450 system, and it can theoretically reduce the effectiveness of oral contraceptives. It has also been approved for use in shift work sleep disorder and for patients with obstructive sleep apnea whose sleepiness persists despite the use of continuous positive airway pressure.

Mild cataplexy often responds to medications that improve alertness because the phenomenon is facilitated by the presence of drowsiness. The classic anticataplectic medica-

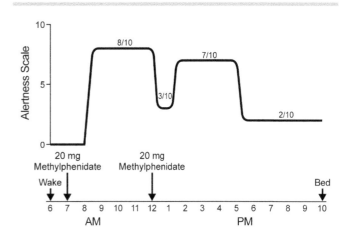

Figure 14 Dose Assessment With Methylphenidate. A visual method can be used to assess the response of patients to drug therapy for narcolepsy. By using a scale of alertness that ranges from 1 to 10 (1=so sleepy the patient is fast asleep; 10=the patient is fully and normally awake), it is possible to determine whether individual doses of stimulants or the frequency of their administration should be increased. In this patient, the second dose should be administered earlier and a third dose should be instituted, perhaps at 3 PM. (Adapted from Silber MH, Krahn LE, Morgenthaler TI. Sleep Medicine in Clinical Practice. New York: Taylor & Francis, 2004. [Used with permission of Mayo Foundation for Medical Education and Research.])

tions are the antidepressants, including tricyclic drugs such as protriptyline, selective serotonin reuptake inhibitors such as sertraline, and combined serotonin and norepinephrine reuptake inhibitors such as venlafaxine. However, side effects,

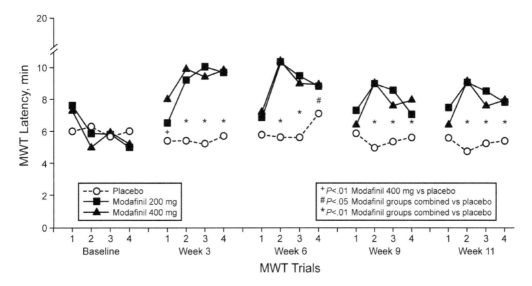

Figure 15 Modafinil for Treatment of Narcolepsy. These graphs illustrate the primary results of a multicenter controlled trial of modafinil in 271 patients with narcolepsy. The maintenance of wakefulness test (MWT) measures the ability of subjects to remain awake while sitting in dim illumination for as long as 40 minutes over four trials in the course of a day. The data show that modafinil results in increased alertness in doses of 200 and 400 mg daily compared with placebo. However, the degree of alertness with the drug is still far below the levels reported for normal subjects (mean, 32.6 minutes). (From US Modafinil in Narcolepsy Multicenter Study Group [31]. [Used with permission.])

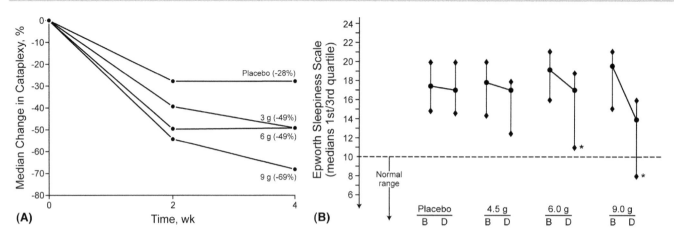

Figure 16 Results of Controlled Trials of Sodium Oxybate for Cataplexy. (A) A multicenter controlled trial of sodium oxybate for the treatment of cataplexy in 136 patients with narcolepsy showed a dose-dependent decrease in the frequency of cataplectic attacks with a clinically significant 69% reduction from baseline at a dose of 9 g per day. (From The US Xyrem Multicenter Study Group. A randomized, double-blind, placebo-controlled multicenter trial comparing the effects of three doses of orally administered sodium oxybate with placebo for the treatment of narcolepsy. Sleep 2002; 25: 42-4. [Used with permission.]) (B) A multicenter controlled trial of adjunctive therapy with sodium oxybate for the treatment of excessive daytime sleepiness in 228 patients with narcolepsy showed significant improvement in the subjective Epworth Sleepiness Scale with 6 g and 9 g per day. Most (78%) patients continued taking other stimulants during the trial. However, the objective maintenance of wakefulness test data (not shown) demonstrated significance at only the 9-g dose. Fifteen of 47 patients (32%) assigned to the 9-g dose discontinued the trial due to adverse events, including nausea, dizziness, and enuresis. B indicates baseline; D, drug. (From Xyrem International Study Group [33]. [Used with permission.])

including weight gain, often limit the use of such anticataplectic medications. More recently, sodium oxybate (γ-hydroxybutyrate), has been found to be highly effective against cataplexy, with reductions of as much as 85% of attacks reported in controlled trials (32). It is administered in liquid form in two doses, the first before sleep and the second 2.5 to 4 hours later. The drug is metabolized in the liver and then excreted as carbon dioxide. Its mechanism of action is undetermined. In addition to its anticataplectic effect, it enhances slow-wave sleep and, at higher doses, increases daytime alertness (Figure 16) (33). However, it is potentially dependence-producing, and its side effects, especially noticeable at high doses, include headache, dizziness, nausea, constipation, nocturnal enuresis, sleepwalking, and nocturnal confusion. It can cause depression of the central nervous system and the respiratory system, and it should not be used in conjunction with alcohol or other sedative hypnotics. It should not be used in patients with untreated sleep apnea, obesity-hypoventilation syndrome, or chronic obstructive pulmonary disease.

Nonpharmacological approaches may be helpful as adjunct therapies or as the sole treatment for patients with mild narcolepsy, especially for those who refrain from driving. Strategic napping for brief periods may subsequently increase alertness for several hours. Judicious use of caffeinated drinks may enhance alertness at those times when it is essential. Many patients with disabling or embarrassing cataplexy learn to control their emotions to avoid spells of muscle weakness.

The autoimmune hypothesis of narcolepsy has led to several attempts at immunosuppressant or immunomodulatory therapy in patients for whom the disease was identified soon after onset. Prednisone, plasmapheresis, and intravenous

immunoglobulin have been used in single reported cases with rather disappointing results. In some patients, the frequency of cataplectic episodes has appeared to decline, but there have been no consistent changes in objective measures such as latency on the multiple sleep latency test or the maintenance of wakefulness test or CSF hcrt-1 concentrations (34–36). To be effective, such therapies may have to be administered at the start of the disease process before the death of any hcrt-synthesizing neurons.

REFERENCES

1. Schenck CH, Bassetti CL, Arnulf I, Mignot E. English Translations of the First Clinical Reports on Narcolepsy by Gélineau and on Cataplexy by Westphal in the Late 19th Century, with Commentary. In: Bassetti CL, Billiard M, Mignot E, editors. Narcolepsy and Hypersomnia. New York: Informa Healthcare, 2007. p. 7–24

2. Longstreth WT Jr, Koepsell TD, Ton TG, Hendrickson AF, van Belle G. The epidemiology of narcolepsy. Sleep 2007; 30: 13–26.

3. Silber MH, Krahn LE, Olson EJ, Pankratz VS. The epidemiology of narcolepsy in Olmsted County, Minnesota: a population-based study. Sleep 2002; 25: 197–202.

4. Moore WR, Silber MH, Decker PA, et al. Cataplexy Emotional Trigger Questionnaire (CETQ): a brief patient screen to identify cataplexy in patients with narcolepsy. J Clin Sleep Med 2007; 3: 37–40.

5. Guilleminault C, Mignot E, Partinen M. Controversies in the diagnosis of narcolepsy. Sleep 1994; 17(8 Suppl):S1–6.

6. Okun ML, Lin L, Pelin Z, Hong S, Mignot E. Clinical aspects of narcolepsy-cataplexy across ethnic groups. Sleep 2002; 25: 27–35.

7. Ohayon MM. Prevalence of hallucinations and their pathological associations in the general population. Psychiatry Res 2000; 97: 153–64.

8. Ohayon MM, Zulley J, Guilleminault C, Smirne S. Prevalence and pathologic associations of sleep paralysis in the general population. Neurology 1999; 52: 1194–200.

9. Silber MH, Krahn LE, Slocumb NL. Clinical and polysomnographic findings of narcolepsy with and without cataplexy: a population-based study [abstract]. Sleep 2003; 26(Suppl): A282–3.

10. Kotagal S, Krahn LE, Slocumb N. A putative link between childhood narcolepsy and obesity. Sleep Med 2004; 5: 147–50.

11. Vogel G. Studies in psychophysiology of dreams. III. The dream of narcolepsy. Arch Gen Psychiatry 1960; 3: 421–8.

12. Juji T, Satake M, Honda Y, Doi Y. HLA antigens in Japanese patients with narcolepsy: all the patients were DR2 positive. Tissue Antigens 1984; 24: 316–9.

13. Mignot E, Hayduk R, Black J, Grumet FC, Guilleminault C. HLA DQB1*0602 is associated with cataplexy in 509 narcoleptic patients. Sleep 1997; 20: 1012–20.

14. Mignot E. Genetic and familial aspects of narcolepsy. Neurology 1998; 50(2 Suppl 1): S16–22.

15. Black JL 3rd, Krahn LE, Pankratz VS, Silber M. Search for neuron-specific and nonneuron-specific antibodies in narcoleptic patients with and without HLA DQB1*0602. Sleep 2002; 25: 719–23.

16. Black JL 3rd, Silber MH, Krahn LE, et al. Analysis of hypocretin (orexin) antibodies in patients with narcolepsy. Sleep 2005; 28: 427–31.

17. Smith AJ, Jackson MW, Neufing P, McEvoy RD, Gordon TP. A functional autoantibody in narcolepsy. Lancet 2004; 364: 2122–4.

18. Black JL 3rd, Avula RK, Walker DL, et al. HLA DQB1*0602 positive narcoleptic subjects with cataplexy have CSF IgG reactive to rat hypothalamic protein extract. Sleep 2005; 28: 1191–2.

19. Hallmayer J, Faraco J, Lin L, et al. Narcolepsy is strongly associated with the T-cell receptor alpha locus. Nat Genet 2009; 41: 708–11. Epub 2009 May 3. Erratum in: Nat Genet 2009; 41: 859.

20. Aran A, Lin L, Nevsimalova S, et al. Elevated anti-streptococcal antibodies in patients with recent narcolepsy onset. Sleep 2009; 32: 979–83.

21. Lin L, Faraco J, Li R, et al. The sleep disorder canine narcolepsy is caused by a mutation in the hypocretin (orexin) receptor 2 gene. Cell 1999; 98: 365–76.

22. Chemelli RM, Willie JT, Sinton CM, et al. Narcolepsy in orexin knockout mice: molecular genetics of sleep regulation. Cell 1999; 98: 437–51.

23. Ripley B, Overeem S, Fujiki N, et al. CSF hypocretin/orexin levels in narcolepsy and other neurological conditions. Neurology 2001; 57: 2253–8.

24. Thannickal TC, Moore RY, Nienhuis R, et al. Reduced number of hypocretin neurons in human narcolepsy. Neuron 2000; 27: 469–74.

25. Malik S, Boeve BF, Krahn LE, Silber MH. Narcolepsy associated with other central nervous system disorders. Neurology 2001; 57: 539–41.

26. AASM. The International Classification of Sleep Disorders: Diagnostic and Coding Manual. 2nd ed. Westchester (IL): American Academy of Sleep Medicine, 2005.

27. Anderson KN, Pilsworth S, Sharples LD, Smith IE, Shneerson JM. Idiopathic hypersomnia: a study of 77 cases. Sleep 2007; 30: 1274–81.

28. Littner M, Johnson SF, McCall WV, et al; Standards of Practice Committee. Practice parameters for the treatment of narcolepsy: an update for 2000. Sleep 2001; 24: 451–66.

29. Auger RR, Goodman SH, Silber MH, Krahn LE, Pankratz VS, Slocumb NL. Risks of high-dose stimulants in the treatment of disorders of excessive somnolence: a case-control study. Sleep 2005; 28: 667–72.

30. US Modafinil in Narcolepsy Multicenter Study Group. Randomized trial of modafinil for the treatment of pathological somnolence in narcolepsy. Ann Neurol 1998; 43: 88–97.

31. US Modafinil in Narcolepsy Multicenter Study Group. Randomized trial of modafinil as a treatment for the excessive daytime somnolence of narcolepsy: Neurology 2000; 54: 1166–75.

32. Xyrem International Study Group. Further evidence supporting the use of sodium oxybate for the treatment of cataplexy: a double-blind, placebo-controlled study in 228 patients. Sleep Med 2005; 6: 415–21.

33. Xyrem International Study Group. A double-blind, placebo-controlled study demonstrates sodium oxybate is effective for the treatment of excessive daytime sleepiness in narcolepsy. J Clin Sleep Med 2005; 1: 391–7.

34. Fronczek R, Verschuuren J, Lammers GJ. Response to intravenous immunoglobulins and placebo in a patient with narcolepsy with cataplexy. J Neurol 2007; 254: 1607–8. Epub 2007 Sep 4.

35. Plazzi G, Poli F, Franceschini C, et al. Intravenous high-dose immunoglobulin treatment in recent onset childhood narcolepsy with cataplexy. J Neurol 2008; 255: 1549–54. Epub 2008 Sep 3.

36. Valko PO, Khatami R, Baumann CR, Bassetti CL. No persistent effect of intravenous immunoglobulins in patients with narcolepsy with cataplexy. J Neurol 2008; 255: 1900–3. Epub 2008 Sep 25.

8

Insomnia

Lois E. Krahn, MD

ABBREVIATIONS

FDG, [^{18}F]fluorodeoxyglucose

GABA, γ-aminobutyric acid

ICSD-2, *International Classification of Sleep Disorders: Diagnostic and Coding Manual,* 2nd edition

NREM, non–rapid eye movement

PET, positron emission tomography

REM, rapid eye movement

Insomnia, the most common sleep disorder, causes distress to millions of people worldwide. The *International Classification of Sleep Disorders: Diagnostic and Coding Manual* (2nd ed [ICSD-2]) (1) defines insomnia as the inability to fall asleep or stay asleep or the experience of only unrefreshing sleep, with the result that one's daytime functioning is compromised (Figure 1). Insomnia cannot be defined simply in terms of the number of hours of sleep missed. This important point arises in clinical practice because some patients seek treatment out of concern that they are not sleeping eight hours a night. No universally accepted minimum sleep duration has been established because there is considerable interindividual variability. Some persons (<5%) are short sleepers, as defined by the ICSD-2, and they function well day after day on five hours of sleep or less (1). No existing sleep test can affirm the optimum amount of sleep to help distinguish between a patient with insomnia and a patient who is a short sleeper. The most important diagnostic step is for the clinician to ascertain that the patient experiences some degree of daytime impairment because of unsatisfactory sleep.

The two extremes of the sleep spectrum range from excessive time in bed to insufficient sleep syndrome. Patients who overestimate their sleep needs can aggravate their sleep problem by allocating excessive time for sleep (Figure 2). This mismatch may result in undesired wakefulness relative to the person's sleep expectations. In these cases, inadequate sleep hygiene is commonly a major contributor to insomnia. Patient education that helps individual patients develop an awareness of their functioning, including drowsiness and alertness, allows them to gauge their preferred bedtime and awakening times. Underestimating the amount of sleep achieved and excessively restricting the patient's time in bed may lead to daytime fatigue (but not to nighttime wakefulness).

MECHANISMS OF INSOMNIA

Insomnia has numerous causes (Figure 3). In clinical practice, chronic insomnia is not due to a single etiologic factor but instead has multiple intertwined mechanisms, both physiolog-

ical and psychological. A valuable model of chronic insomnia proposed by Spielman (2) conceptualizes three components: vulnerability, triggers, and a perpetuating process. For example, physiologically a patient may be a lifelong "light sleeper" with an increased risk of insomnia because of heightened baseline levels of central nervous system arousal. After a psychologically stressful event triggers insomnia, the sleeplessness is then sustained by environmental factors, behavioral issues, or concurrent illnesses. An alternate approach is to classify insomnia into primary and secondary types by whether a cause of the sleep disruption can be identified. However, this more simplistic scheme does not reflect the complexity of insomnia nor does it identify to the same degree the perpetuating conditions that could eventually be addressed in a treatment plan. The nosology for insomnia that was adopted in 2005 by ICSD-2 will be discussed in more detail later in this chapter.

Physiological Vulnerability

Persons may be vulnerable physiologically to insomnia for various reasons. In isolation, the precondition is not sufficient to produce insomnia but it does provide a substrate that is conducive to sleeplessness in the context of other factors. Recognizing the perpetuating conditions is useful in predicting which patients will be at higher risk of relapse and who might benefit from continuing therapy.

Heightened Central Nervous System Arousal

When wakefulness is sustained, the pressure to fall asleep builds. This phenomenon, called homeostatic pressure, is a linear relationship as long as the individual has a consistent sleep-wake schedule or, in other words, an entrained circadian rhythm of sleep. Underdeveloped homeostatic pressure is a potential mechanism for insomnia, although this factor must always be considered within the context of the sleep-wake circadian rhythm. In cases of jet lag or shift work sleep disorder, a misaligned body clock significantly interferes with the capacity for homeostatic pressure to mount.

Recent neuroimaging studies have looked for evidence of an increased level of arousal in patients with insomnia by using [^{18}F]fluorodeoxyglucose (FDG) positron emission tomography (PET) to test the hypothesis that patients with insomnia have a higher whole-brain metabolic rate while awake and during non–rapid eye movement (NREM) sleep (Figure 4) (3). The hypothesis is that the metabolic rate of wake-promoting brain structures does not decline sufficiently from wake to sleep states in patients with insomnia. Consequently, daytime fatigue is associated with reductions in wake metabolism in thalamocortical networks, especially the prefrontal cortex. Preliminary PET data confirmed the presence of higher rates of cerebral metabolism during the NREM sleep of insomnia patients.

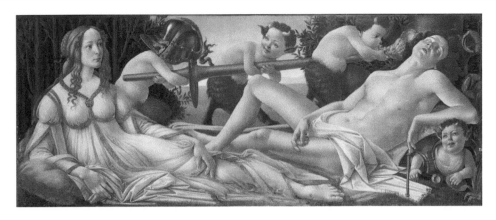

Figure 1 *Venus and Mars* by Sandro Botticelli (Tempura and Oil on Poplar; Circa 1485). Sleep and its disruption have been depicted in paintings throughout the centuries. (From National Gallery, London/Art Resource, New York. [Used with permission.]).

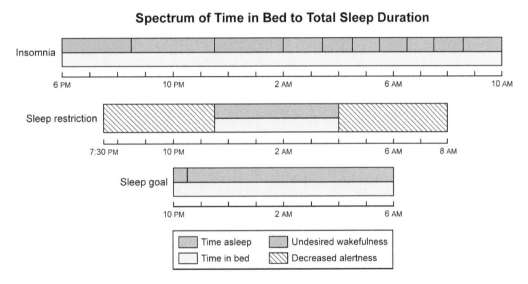

Figure 2 Spectrum of Time in Bed to Total Sleep Duration. The two extremes of the sleep spectrum range from excessive time asleep in bed to insufficient sleep syndrome.

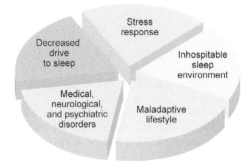

Figure 3 Possible Mechanisms of Insomnia. The key factors contributing to insomnia are predisposition, stress, environment, lifestyle, and medical disorders.

Nofzinger et al. (3) theorized that these observations may be due to less reduction in activity in subcortical structures during the transition from wake to sleep compared with that of healthy controls. They furthermore speculated that neural networks exist in the neurobiology of insomnia, including a general arousal system (ascending reticular formation and hypothalamus), a cognitive system (prefrontal cortex), and an emotion-regulating system (hippocampus, amygdala, and anterior cingulate cortex) (3).

Neurochemical imbalances, such as a deficit of inhibitory neurotransmitters or an excess of stimulating ones, may cause a state of chronic hyperarousal (4). To date, sparse research data support this theory. Nonetheless, the theory that underdeveloped homeostatic pressure contributes to insomnia is plausible in view of the recent finding that hypocretin deficiency plays a critical role in the mechanism of narcolepsy, a disorder of excessive daytime sleepiness. The absence or excess of a

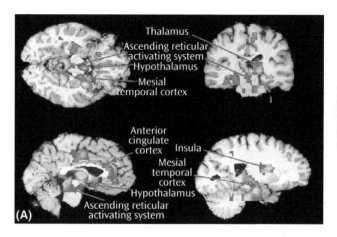

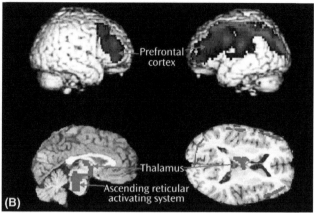

Figure 4 Positron Emission Tomography Scans of the Brain of a Patient With Insomnia. (A) A patient with insomnia who is in non–rapid eye movement (NREM) sleep has less change than controls in relative metabolism during the transition from awake to NREM sleep as measured by regional glucose metabolism. (B) A patient with insomnia who is awake has reduced activity (compared to that in controls) in the frontal cortex bilaterally, in the left hemisphere and thalamus, and in the hypothalamus and brainstem reticular formation. These changes may represent subjective daytime fatigue. (From Nofzinger et al. [3]. [Used with permission.])

neurochemical factor (or factors) that contributes to disorders of excessive wakefulness is certainly possible. However, the lack of a highly specific phenotype of insomnia, as exists in the case of narcolepsy with cataplexy, has hampered research efforts.

Genetic Factors
The degree to which genetic factors predispose a person to insomnia is little understood. The ICSD-2 standardized outline uses the category of familial pattern for each recognized subtype of insomnia but cites little research. A positive family history of insomnia has been reported in 73% of patients with insomnia compared with 24% in controls (5). The responsible genes are still largely unknown. Described mechanisms include a point mutation in the prion protein gene (*PRNP*) that causes a rare disease called *fatal familial insomnia* and a missense mutation of the gene responsible for the GABA (γ-aminobutyric acid) subunit $GABA_A$ β_3 (6).

Triggers

Patients with insomnia often describe sleep of acceptable duration and quality up to a discrete point in time when something triggers disturbed sleep. The insomnia evaluation traditionally focuses on the identification of the trigger. The precipitants of insomnia can be subdivided into two main categories: 1) external circumstances (e.g., a new lawsuit) or 2) internal experiences (e.g., catastrophic thinking) (Table 1).

External Circumstances
Tremendous interindividual variability exists regarding which events are stressful, to which degree a person perceives these events as threatening, and whether emotional distress or tension results in disrupted sleep.

Many persons experience difficulty sleeping from time to time when their coping mechanisms are overwhelmed by stress. Emotionally charged events can be either negative (e.g., an ill parent) or positive (e.g., an upcoming family wed-

Table 1 Events that may trigger insomnia

Type of circumstance	Events
External circumstances	Loss or bereavement
	Relationship breakup
	Relocation
	Career transitions (termination or initiation)
	Examinations
	Health concerns
	Financial challenges (mortgage, pension, investments)
	Regulatory concerns (tax returns or audit)
	Legal problems (lawsuit)
Internal experiences	Catastrophic thinking
	Lack of control over circumstances
	Fear of the unknown
	Loneliness
	Boredom
	Uncertainty regarding direction in life
	Perfectionism
	Low self-esteem
	Suppressed emotions

ding). Individuals vary in their capacity to handle stress. Routine events, such as a looming tax deadline, can be a substantial source of worry and tension for some persons, whereas others view them as just another mundane task. Persons susceptible to stress, many of whom have an obsessive personality type or a history of trauma, amplify the necessary preparation for, or the possible consequences of, an event. In so doing, they escalate their stress level, which leads to heightened muscle tension and poorer sleep (Figure 5). Not everyone is vulnerable to stress-related insomnia. In contrast, some persons crave excitement and consciously seek out stressful careers (e.g., firefighting) or

Influence of Stress in Patients With Insomnia

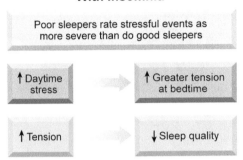

Figure 5 Influence of Stress in Patients With Insomnia. Stress contributes to increased tension and initial insomnia.

Factors Contributing to Development and Persistence of Insomnia

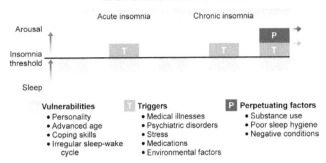

Figure 6 Factors Contributing to Development and Perpetuation of Insomnia. Insomnia has a multifactorial basis.

extreme leisure activities (e.g., skydiving) because they thrive on unpredictable and emotionally demanding situations. These persons have a higher threshold for perceiving an event as stressful and also do not experience the sustained muscle tension that interferes with sleep. The absence of a diathesis that confers a vulnerability for insomnia may play a protective function as well.

Internal Experiences

Only insomnia that evolves into chronic disease is typically brought to the attention of medical providers. Whatever precipitated the sleeplessness may have occurred months or years earlier. The insomnia may have taken on a life of its own and may no longer be linked directly to the past trigger. Other conditions emerge and exert influence over time that maintain the ongoing process. Both the trigger and the perpetuating process may stem from a common source, such as anxiety; for example, initially time-limited anticipatory anxiety related to an upcoming event may be followed by generalized anxiety that persists over time. In the absence of enduring anxiety, the sleep loss would likely be more limited in duration.

Perpetuating Process

Three conditions that compromise sleep quality are 1) environments that are not conducive to restful sleep, 2) behaviors and attitudes of the sleeper that prove to be maladaptive, and 3) underlying psychiatric or medical disorders. These problems can function both as the initial trigger for the onset of insomnia and, if ongoing, as sustainers of the process. Figure 6 depicts how chronic insomnia develops when there is convergence of the three components of predisposition, triggers, and perpetuating process.

Inhospitable Environment

A wide array of circumstances can be disruptive to sleep (Table 2), including the actions of other persons (Figure 7) or an unsettling sleep environment (Figure 8). When persons travel, for example, they recognize that they may have to sleep temporarily under less-than-desirable circumstances and they are usually well aware that the quality of their sleep will suffer. However, other sleep

Table 2 Environmental conditions associated with insomnia

Environmental condition	Examples
Noise	Snoring
	Coughing
	Music; television
	Traffic
	Telephone; pager
	Child or adult seeking attention
	Burglar, car, and other alarms
	Mechanical sounds (e.g., elevator in motion or ticking clock)
	Barking dog
Light	Bright light (e.g., during summer at extreme latitudes or because of shift work)
Movement	Vibration (e.g., while traveling by airplane or car)
	Body movement (e.g., thrashing about by bed partner)
	Pets
Foods	Heartburn; gastroesophageal reflux disease
	Bloating; excessive gas
Extreme temperatures	Heat (e.g., lack of air conditioning)
	Cold (e.g., insufficient bedcovers)
Bedding materials	Uncomfortable bed
	Hard pillow
	Allergies to laundry soap, fabric softeners, or feathers

environments less conducive to sleep that are more enduring may be less obvious. Patients may underestimate the degree to which familiar and accepted environmental conditions contribute to insomnia. Notable examples are the cultural practices that influence sleeping arrangements. Beds, bedding materials, and the number of other sleepers in the bed may vary, with subcultures maintaining traditions in which a good quality of sleep may not be the highest priority (Figure 9). A snoring bed partner or the proximity of pets can also compromise sleep quality (Figure 10).

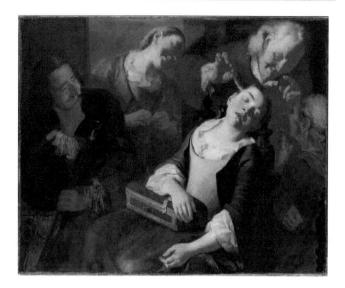

Figure 7 *Teasing a Sleeping Girl* by Gaspare Traversi (Oil on Canvas; Circa 1750). Poor quality sleep may be due to environmental factors, including body position or disruptive people or animals. (From The Metropolitan Museum of Art/Art Resource, New York. [Used with permission.])

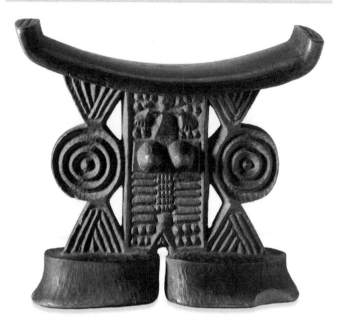

Figure 9 African Wooden Pillow. Nineteenth-century wooden headrests such as this one (16 cm [about 6.5 inches] high) were made by the Shona carvers of Zimbabwe and used mainly by men who were thought to be visiting their ancestors during sleep. (From The Trustees of the British Museum, London. [Used with permission.])

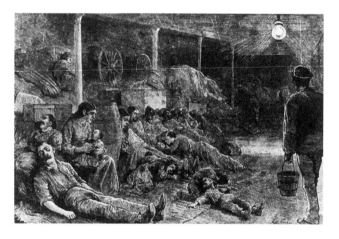

Figure 8 Crowded Sleeping Conditions During Nineteenth-Century River Travel. In this print made from a wood engraving (circa 1875), John Maynard Woodward aptly conveys the crowded conditions on a Mississippi River steamboat filled with men, women, and children deck passengers. (From U.S. National Library of Medicine, Bethesda, MD.)

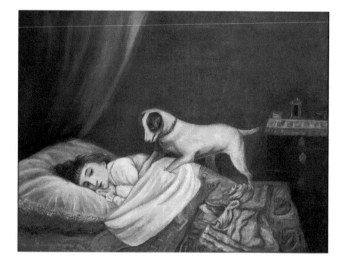

Figure 10 A Sleeping Child Being Disturbed by a Dog. The sleep environment may be disruptive to quality of sleep because of the activity of companion animals. (*Sleeping Child With Dog*; Convent of St. Joseph's, St. Louis, MO; 1886) (From Girard Foundation Collection. Museum of International Folk Art (DCA), Sante Fe, NM. Photo by Blair Clark. [Used with permission.])

Potentially Maladaptive Behaviors and Attitudes

Table 3 lists behaviors and attitudes that can lead to acute insomnia becoming a chronic disorder. The cognitive experiences that serve as triggers of insomnia may also perpetuate the process. An inconsistent sleep-wake schedule is a common cause of insomnia (Figure 11). Some patients have long-standing insights into the thoughts and behaviors that fuel their insomnia, yet they have been incapable of changing them.

Other patients at the onset of a sleep evaluation have only a limited awareness and recognition of the contributing factors.

Psychiatric and Medical Disorders

Medical conditions, such as clinically significant gastroesophageal reflux disease, can contribute to insomnia, as can

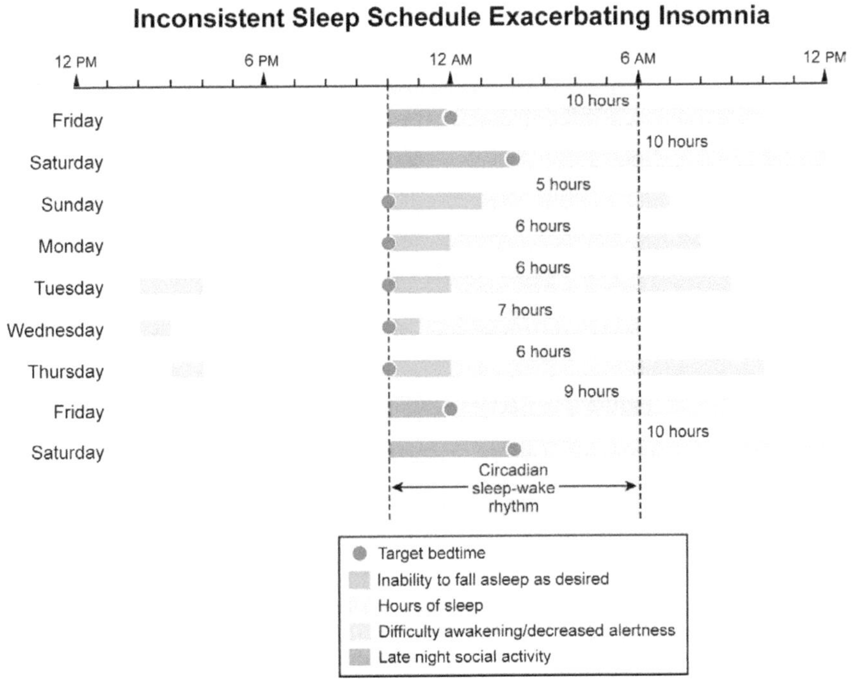

Inconsistent Sleep Schedule Exacerbating Insomnia

Figure 11 Inconsistent Sleep Schedule Exacerbating Insomnia. An inconsistent sleep-wake schedule can have a disruptive effect on the timing of sleep.

Table 3 Lifestyle issues that may compromise sleep

Lifestyle issues
Demanding schedules filled with physically or mentally stimulating activity right up to bedtime
Mind and body unprepared at bedtime to drift off to sleep
Using the bed for activities other than sleep or physical intimacy (e.g., paying bills, reading mail, or using laptop computer)
Increasingly frustrating thought patterns when unable to fall asleep promptly
Heightened muscle tension after failing to fall asleep promptly
Anticipating difficulty falling asleep hours before bedtime
Reduced confidence in ability to fall asleep
Frequent checking of bedside clock
Switching to potentially stimulating activities (e.g., browsing the Internet, watching television, or doing housework) or worrying when unable to sleep
Inconsistent sleep-wake schedule
Excessive use of caffeine
Use of alcohol as sleep aid
Inadequate physical exercise or sedentary lifestyle

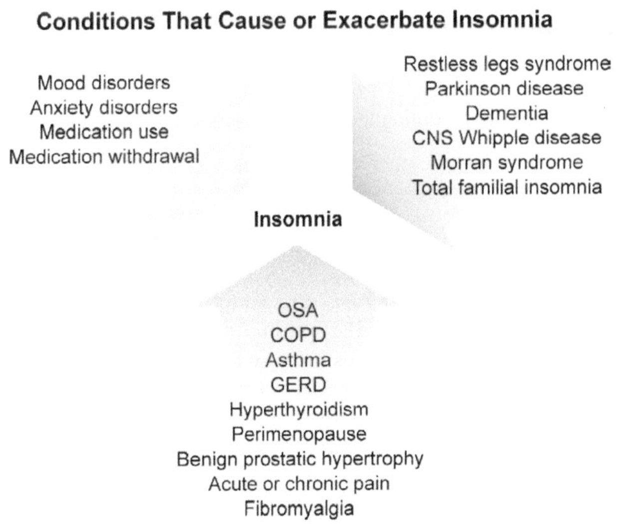

Conditions That Cause or Exacerbate Insomnia

Figure 12 Conditions That Cause or Exacerbate Insomnia. A wide range of conditions is associated with insomnia. CNS, central nervous system; COPD, chronic obstructive pulmonary disease; GERD, gastroesophageal reflux disease; OSA, obstructive sleep apnea.

psychiatric conditions, such as generalized anxiety disorder. A multitude of conditions, from associated illnesses (Figure 12) to associated psychiatric disorders (Table 4), can lead to complaints of insomnia.

Insomnia at Perimenopause

Perimenopausal sleep disruption provides an excellent example of insomnia's multifactorial nature. Compared with the rate of insomnia in premenopausal women, the rate of insomnia in women undergoing the perimenopausal transition is increased dramatically (Figure 13). Thus the risk of chronic insomnia increases as women age, especially when the trigger and the

perpetuating process coexist in a woman with a premenopausal predisposition toward insomnia.

By examining this example more closely, we can see that multiple risk factors play a role in insomnia that develops at perimenopause; these risk factors include ones that cannot be modified (e.g., being female and undergoing the aging process)

Table 4 Sleep disturbances due to psychiatric disorders

Sleep disturbance	Psychiatric disorders
Insomnia	Major depression
	Dysthymia
	Manic phase
	Hypomanic phase
	Posttraumatic stress disorder
	Acute stress disorder
	Generalized anxiety disorder
	Panic disorder
	Somatization disorder
	Chronic pain secondary to psychological factors
	Schizophrenia
	Attention deficit disorder with hyperactivity
Nightmares	Posttraumatic stress disorder

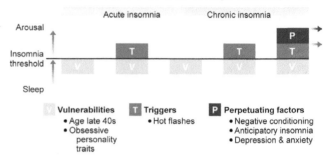

Factors Contributing to Development and Persistence of Insomnia During Perimenopause

Figure 14 Factors Contributing to Development and Perpetuation of Insomnia During Perimenopause. Women at highest risk of insomnia during perimenopause have a combination of vulnerable preconditions, triggering events, and perpetuating factors.

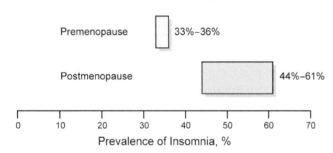

Insomnia in Perimenopause

Figure 13 Insomnia in Perimenopause. Sleep disruptions often increase in women during the time just before and after menopause.

and others that can often be altered with therapy (e.g., hot flashes, anxiety, depressed mood, thyroid insufficiency, and increased upper airway resistance). Hot flashes, widely recognized as a cause of sleep disruption during the perimenopausal transition, are abrupt surges in body temperature that can lead to bouts of sweating. The typical hot flash lasts about 3 minutes. The patient is awakened either by warmth or the subsequent chill related to damp clothing and bedding. Hot flashes are precipitated by declines in estrogen levels that signal a narrowing of the thermoregulatory zone of the hypothalamus, which has a diminished capacity to adapt to a wide range of ambient temperatures. The neurotransmitters serotonin and norepinephrine are believed to play secondary roles in this thermo-

regulatory control pathway. Perimenopausal insomnia can be exacerbated by anxiety. Women who feel anxious have been found to have more hot flashes than control subjects (7). The three-component multifactorial model aptly illustrates the issues at play in this example of insomnia and points toward potential targets of therapy (Figure 14).

SUBTYPES OF INSOMNIA

The National Sleep Foundation conducts annual surveys in the United States (8) to examine the epidemiology of sleep disorders using a scheme that classifies insomnia by the duration of symptoms. The 2002 community survey conducted by the National Sleep Foundation documented that most respondents (58%) reported having insomnia at least a few nights a month (Figure 15) (8).

There has been an attempt in ICSD-2 to be more precise in the approach to insomnia (Table 5). A more specific conceptualization of insomnia is particularly important for research purposes because observations about the epidemiology, etiology, natural history, and treatment of sleeplessness may apply only to distinctive subsets of patients who share similar characteristics. Subdividing insomnia has been challenging because of limited clinical and laboratory data about the possible subtypes and causes. Focusing on the interplay of vulnerabilities, triggering events, and the perpetuating process of insomnia can be useful in understanding the differences between insomnia subtypes (Figure 16).

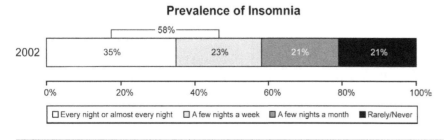

Prevalence of Insomnia

Figure 15 Prevalence of Insomnia. Data from the 2002 National Sleep Foundation survey showed that most respondents reported insomnia. (From National Sleep Foundation. [Used with permission.])

Table 5 ICSD-2 subtypes of insomnia

Subtype	Prevalence in general population, %	Onset	Duration	Primary mechanism	Vulnerabilities	Triggers	Perpetuating process
Adjustment (acute, short-term, or transient)	15–20	Acute	<3 months	Stress	Increased age, female sex, history of light sleep, anxiety, obsessive thinking, depressed mood	Specific stressor (positive or negative life event)	Unknown
Psychophysiological insomnia (conditioned insomnia)	1–2	Acute or gradual	Chronic	Maladaptive sleep behaviors, stress (about falling asleep)	Female sex, anxiety, obsessive thinking	Variable	Negative thought patterns and increased muscle tension at bedtime
Paradoxical insomnia (sleep state misperception; severe insomnia without objective evidence of any sleep disturbance)	Unknown but likely rare	Unknown	Variable from months to years	Unknown	Unknown	Unknown	Unknown
Idiopathic insomnia (childhood-onset insomnia)	0.7–1	Childhood	Chronic	Increased CNS arousal	Unknown; minimization of interpersonal issues	None known	Unknown
Inadequate sleep hygiene	1–2 in adults <30 years of age	Unknown but likely gradual	Chronic	Environmental factors, maladaptive sleep behaviors	Younger age, poor knowledge of healthy sleep habits	Unknown	Poor sleep hygiene, use of caffeine and other substances
Behavioral insomnia of childhood (sleep onset association disorder)	10–30	Not before age 6 months	Unknown	Maladaptive sleep behaviors	Demanding temperament, caretakers' behaviors, active medical disorder	Unknown	Caretakers' behaviors
Insomnia due to drugs or substances	0.2	Any age	Variable	Alcohol, stimulants, excessive use of caffeine, hypnotic withdrawal, food allergy, toxins	None specifically	Substance abuse	None specifically
Insomnia due to psychiatric disorder	3	Any age	Variable	Anxiety, depression, bipolar disorder	Female sex, younger age	Psychiatric disorder	None specifically
Insomnia due to medical disorder	Unknown	Any age	Variable	Hot flashes, night sweats, dyspnea, wheezing, coughing	None specifically	Medical disorder	None specifically

Abbreviations: CNS, central nervous system; ICSD-2, *International Classification of Sleep Disorders: Diagnostic and Coding Manual*, 2nd edition; NA, not available.
Data from *The International Classification of Sleep Disorders: Diagnostic and Coding Manual* (1). Used with permission.

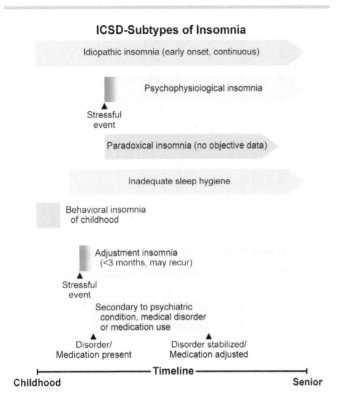

ICSD-Subtypes of Insomnia

Idiopathic insomnia (early onset, continuous)

Psychophysiological insomnia

Stressful
event

Paradoxical insomnia (no objective data)

Inadequate sleep hygiene

Behavioral insomnia
of childhood

Adjustment insomnia
(<3 months, may recur)

Stressful
event

Secondary to psychiatric
condition, medical disorder
or medication use

Disorder/   Disorder stabilized/
Medication present   Medication adjusted

—————— Timeline ——————
Childhood   Senior

Figure 16 ICSD-2 Subtypes of Insomnia. Subtypes of insomnia vary by age of onset and natural course. ICSD-2, *International Classification of Sleep Disorders: Diagnostic and Coding Manual*, 2nd edition.

DIAGNOSIS OF INSOMNIA

Obtaining a comprehensive sleep history from the patient is the pivotal component of an insomnia evaluation. The clinician needs to gain an in-depth understanding of the patient's sleep over time by covering all the components discussed in the preceding section that could be producing unsatisfactory sleep. The clinician should strive to determine the relative importance of the identified factors and whether they might be modified with treatment.

Other diagnostic tools may also be used to augment the comprehensive sleep history (Table 6); however, these should never be viewed as a substitute for the sleep history. The diagnosis of insomnia does not depend on the presence of any particular physiological event. Consequently, polysomnography has only a limited role as a diagnostic tool in the assessment of patients with insomnia (9). Sleep studies are difficult to conduct because sleeping in a sleep laboratory causes a subset of patients with insomnia to experience increased muscle tension and anxiety. The experience of being observed or of having

to wear multiple monitors can further inhibit the ability to drift off to sleep. In contrast, a paradoxical response has also been described (10). Patients who struggle to fall sleep and stay asleep in the familiar setting of home are more relaxed and sleepy in a sleep disorders center. This phenomenon illustrates the negative conditioning whereby a familiar setting can prevent the mental and muscle relaxation necessary for a rapid transition from wakefulness to sleep.

Polysomnography is indicated as a diagnostic test for patients with insomnia when their sleeplessness exists in the context of other suspected sleep disorders. When snoring, apnea, or unusual behaviors are present, sleep studies conducted in a sleep laboratory can be invaluable. After determining that another sleep disorder is present, the clinician can decide whether to treat it before treating the insomnia or to treat them both currently if the insomnia is of sufficient severity to merit a concurrent approach.

With the subtype of insomnia called *paradoxical insomnia*, polysomnography aids in establishing the diagnosis. Patients with this condition seek care for sleeplessness that seems disproportionate to the objective findings. The insomnia typically persists despite treatment trials of behavioral and pharmacologic approaches. Family members may be able to offer observations about whether the patient appears to sleep at some points during the night. In this situation, a sleep study can reveal whether the patient is sleeping better than indicated by self-report. These data can refocus efforts away from trials of hypnotic agents and instead lead to an exploration of whether anxiety is causing the patient to amplify the insomnia.

Physiological assessment is an additional tool available in select sleep disorders centers. Drifting off to sleep is difficult when a patient is wound up tightly and has a high level of physiological arousal. Surface measurements of the muscle tone and the skin temperature of the forehead can help discriminate between tense and relaxed states. Biofeedback assessments of this type are typically conducted by psychologists but are not standard practice in many sleep disorders centers. Sensors that show ongoing hyperarousal, even as patients endeavor to relax, indicate that the patient has insufficient relaxation skills or a high baseline level of tension. These observations are not necessary but can be most helpful in establishing the diagnosis of psychophysiological insomnia, particularly when patients overestimate their ability to relax.

The diagnostic algorithm for insomnia (Figure 17) indicates how the sleep history and other diagnostic tools can be used to work through the differential diagnosis.

TREATMENT OF INSOMNIA

Numerous treatment options have been developed to aid patients with insomnia. Clinicians should investigate whether a medical, psychiatric, or substance disorder is a trigger or a perpetuating process or both. When insomnia is secondary to

Table 6 Diagnostic tools for evaluating patients with insomnia

Type of diagnostic tool	Characteristics
Comprehensive sleep history	Interview, sometimes supplemented by questionnaires, collecting a wide range of data
Sleep diary	Detailed prospective account of sleep schedule completed daily by patient
Wrist actigraphy	Compact portable motion detector to measure limb movement
Polysomnography	Test used selectively to confirm whether insomnia is secondary to sleep-disordered breathing
Physiological assessment	Surface frontalis muscle electromyography and skin temperature measurement to gauge degree of relaxation (used in specialized sleep disorders centers)

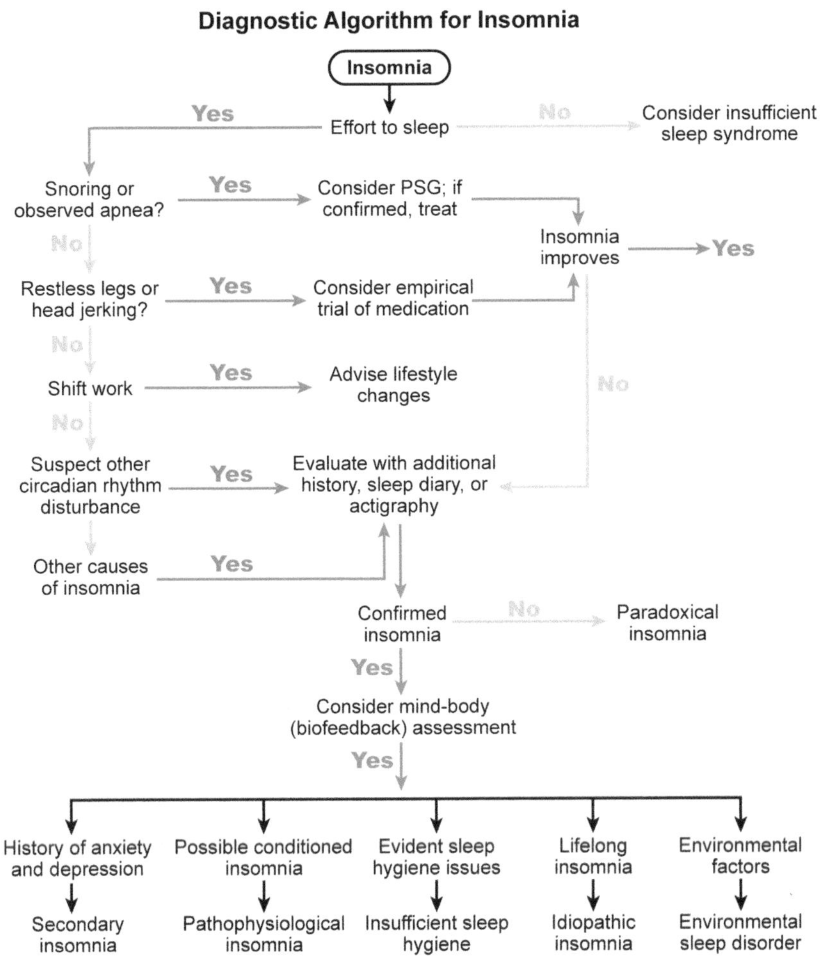

Diagnostic Algorithm for Insomnia

Figure 17 Diagnostic Algorithm for Insomnia. The differential diagnosis of insomnia requires numerous diagnostic steps. PSG, polysomnogram.

Table 7 Basic principles of good sleep hygiene for patients with insomnia

Principle	Actions
Attend to general sleep hygiene	Make getting adequate sleep a priority; strive for consistent sleep-wake schedule
Optimize sleep environment	Eliminate disruptive elements (e.g., pets or noise)
Enhance bedtime routines	Adopt bedtime rituals that aid the relaxing process (e.g., grooming, reading light material, meditation, or listening to soothing music)
Minimize nighttime awakenings	Limit caffeine use; prevent gastroesophageal reflux; avoid excessive exercise close to bedtime; cover up clock face; if awake, do not start stimulating activities (e.g., chores or E-mail)

another condition, a stepwise therapeutic approach can optimize treatment of the overarching primary disorder to whatever degree possible. As a subsequent step, treatment may be used that specifically targets the symptom of insomnia; for example, a hypnotic medication may be prescribed. The clinician should also keep in mind that some insomnia treatments have the potential to aggravate the primary condition. For example, physically demanding yoga techniques may aggravate musculoskeletal pain and benzodiazepines may diminish ventilation in patients with severe chronic obstructive pulmonary disease.

Sleep Education and Hygiene

Patient education about the importance of sleep is an essential part of every treatment plan for insomnia. Health education in U.S. schools historically has not focused on the role played by good quality sleep in overall health. Teaching patients how to achieve good sleep is a key aspect of patient education (Table 7).

Sleep education overlaps with sleep hygiene, a term which refers to the lifestyle choices that influence sleep patterns. Patient education and counseling about optimal sleep hygiene are necessary but often are not sufficient as the sole intervention for patients with insomnia (11). When probing sleep hygiene, clinicians should ask patients to label lifestyle choices as "stimulating" or "relaxing." Patients should be encouraged to consciously participate in activities in the 30 to 60 minutes before going to bed that will help them unwind. Engaging in relaxing, routine behaviors before bedtime is usually beneficial. The focus should be on reinforcing the importance of a regular sleep-wake schedule, with the patient encouraged to have a structured day that includes regular exercise and consistent mealtimes. All subsequent treatments for insomnia will be less effective if sleep hygiene issues are left unaddressed. Optimizing sleep hygiene may be particularly helpful for patients who have sleep-onset insomnia. An effective treatment algorithm (Figure 18) for insomnia builds on the foundation of good sleep education and hygiene.

Nonpharmacologic Treatment

Nonpharmacologic techniques (Table 8) are viewed as the optimal treatment of insomnia, resulting in long-term remission, a sense of mastery for the patient, and no side effects (Figure 19). Several reviews of behavioral techniques for insomnia have examined the efficacy of these techniques (12). The various behavioral treatments have been critically reviewed in a practice parameter published by the American Academy of Sleep Medicine (13). This critical evaluation concluded that stimulus control was the most well-accepted management strategy (Figure 20). Biofeedback, progressive muscle relaxation, and paradoxical intention (i.e., avoiding trying to fall asleep) all have value. Additional useful therapies include sleep restriction (Figure 21)

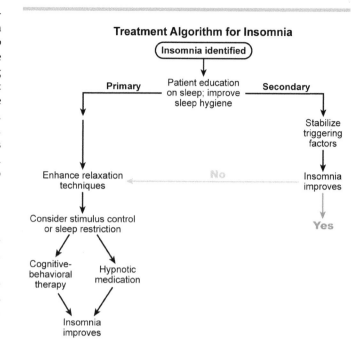

Figure 18 Treatment Algorithm for Insomnia. Treatment of insomnia differs by whether a clear trigger (primary or secondary) can be identified.

Table 8 Recommended behavioral therapies for insomnia

Type of therapy	Implementation techniques
Stimulus control therapy	Reassociate bed with rapid initiation of sleep
Sleep restriction therapy	Reduce time in bed (5-hour minimum) to decrease amount of fragmented sleep
Paradoxical intention	Engage in other relaxing activities instead of trying to fall asleep
Relaxation therapy	Reduce muscle tension to decrease mental arousal; use meditation, hypnosis, imagery training
Cognitive therapy	Identify and modify distorted or catastrophic beliefs about sleep (e.g., a person cannot function after one night of poor-quality sleep)
Biofeedback	Use electromyographic monitoring to reinforce successful relaxation
Multicomponent cognitive-behavioral therapy	Identify and modify attitudes and behaviors unfavorable to sleep

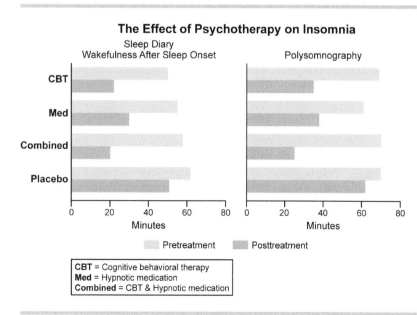

Figure 19 The Effect of Psychotherapy on Insomnia. Psychotherapy is beneficial in treating insomnia whether measured by sleep diary or sleep study. CBT, cognitive-behavioral therapy; combined, cognitive-behavioral therapy and hypnotic medication; med, hypnotic medication.

Stimulus–Control Therapy

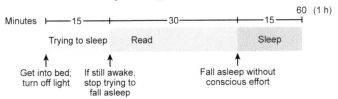

Objective: Associate bed with sleep

- Limit bed to sleep and sexual activity

- Do not use bed for other activities
  (i.e., using laptop, arguing, lounging, or thinking)

- If awake for 15 minutes, stop trying to sleep

- Instead, read a relaxing book or watch
  a calming TV program

Minutes ├────15────┤────────30────────┤────15────┤ 60 (1 h)

Trying to sleep | Read | Sleep

↑ Get into bed; turn off light

↑ If still awake, stop trying to fall asleep

↑ Fall asleep without conscious effort

- Allow your eyelids to get heavy so you can drift off
  to sleep without consciously trying to fall asleep

Figure 20 Stimulus-Control Therapy. The essential element of stimulus-control therapy is not thinking about falling asleep by diverting one's attention to other activities.

Sleep Restriction Therapy

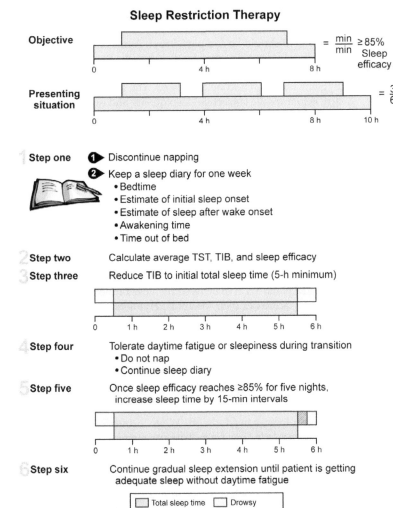

Objective

0   4 h   8 h

$= \dfrac{min}{min} \geq 85\%$ Sleep efficacy

Presenting situation

0   4 h   8 h   10 h

$= \dfrac{360}{600} = 60\%$

Step one ❶ Discontinue napping

❷ Keep a sleep diary for one week
- Bedtime
- Estimate of initial sleep onset
- Estimate of sleep after wake onset
- Awakening time
- Time out of bed

Step two Calculate average TST, TIB, and sleep efficacy

Step three Reduce TIB to initial total sleep time (5-h minimum)

0   1 h   2 h   3 h   4 h   5 h   6 h

Step four Tolerate daytime fatigue or sleepiness during transition
- Do not nap
- Continue sleep diary

Step five Once sleep efficacy reaches ≥85% for five nights, increase sleep time by 15-min intervals

0   1 h   2 h   3 h   4 h   5 h   6 h

Step six Continue gradual sleep extension until patient is getting adequate sleep without daytime fatigue

| Total sleep time | Drowsy |
| Time in bed | Gradual sleep extension |

Figure 21 Sleep Restriction Therapy. Deliberately reducing time in bed aids continuity and quality of sleep. TIB, time in bed; TST, total sleep time.

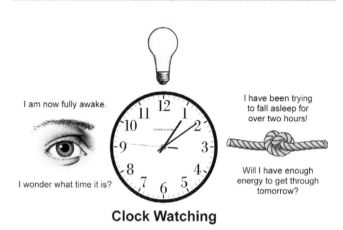

Clock Watching

Figure 22 Clock Watching. Patients with insomnia may focus on the time and worry about its passage while they try to fall asleep.

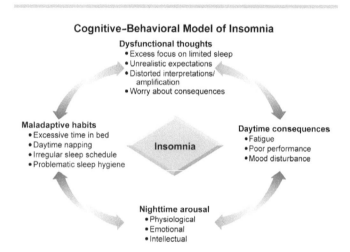

Figure 23 Cognitive-Behavioral Model of Insomnia. Cognitive-behavioral therapy addresses the maladaptive thoughts and habits that perpetuate insomnia.

and cognitive therapy, which concentrates on the maladaptive and distressing thoughts.

Patients who overvalue the role of sleep may fear that going without sufficient sleep for a stretch of time will be lethal. A closely linked perception is that a night of sleeplessness necessarily predicts incurable and enduring sleep problems. Persons with insomnia may also be tempted to monitor the clock during the night to repeatedly verify the exact time, which can serve to escalate their worry about sleeplessness (Figure 22).

Cognitive-behavioral therapy is even more advantageous than pharmacologic treatment in that it addresses both the beliefs and the behaviors that perpetuate insomnia. These include anxiety, lack of confidence in the ability to sleep, and increased muscle tension (14) (Figure 23).

Unfortunately, some patients may have limited access to behavioral therapies. Communities may lack appropriate thera-

Table 9 Relevant characteristics of hypnotic medications

Characteristics
Rate of absorption
Rapidity of distribution to central nervous system
Action on specific neurotransmitters
Duration of elimination half-life
Speed of clearance from central nervous system
Site of metabolism
Presence of active metabolites
Rebound insomnia
Likelihood of tolerance
Risk of dependence

pists or insurance coverage may restrict access to this form of treatment. Thus pharmacologic treatment may be used until a provider of behavioral treatment can be obtained. Whether Internet-based behavioral treatment of insomnia proves effective and fills the relative void in behavioral therapy is being evaluated (15).

Pharmacologic Treatment

General Principles

Sedative hypnotic medications are widely used. Even though starting a sleeping medication may seem straightforward to both the patient and the clinician, a comprehensive sleep assessment should be completed first. A multifaceted treatment plan should precede consideration of any hypnotic (Table 9). Even when it is clear that a medication will be initiated, sleep hygiene issues should be addressed. The goal of hypnotic therapy is to improve subjective sleep quality and quantity, decrease daytime fatigue, improve concentration, and enhance global daytime functioning. Good medical practice calls for using the lowest effective dose for the shortest possible duration. The onset of medication action, which is important for patients with prominent complaints about initial insomnia, is determined by the rate of absorption and distribution. Especially in aging patients or those with hepatic disease, prolonged elimination time increases the risk of excessive sedation, which places patients at increased risk for falls and cognitive impairment.

Hypnotics with longer half-lives also increase the risk of a hangover effect, leading to undesired morning sedation (Figure 24). Some patients interpret morning sleepiness as a need for more sleep and wish to increase the dose of the hypnotic, which instead exacerbates their insomnia. Hypnotics with a short half-life raise a different set of concerns because the sedation can wear off before dawn, leading patients to experience early morning awakenings or rebound insomnia. Triazolam, in particular, has been associated with amnesia. Its relatively high potency and short half-life can cause a patient to awaken abruptly from sleep with residual cognitive impairment.

The challenge of tolerance is another important general pharmacologic consideration. When a medication used long term ceases to induce sleep, patients may increase the dose on their own. Newer agents have been developed to minimize the risks of tolerance and dose escalation. Barbiturates and benzodiazepines are suspected of producing tolerance at a higher rate than do newer medications such as the benzodiazepine receptor agonists. The older agents also can cause physical dependence when patients experience withdrawal symptoms after abrupt discontinuation. The ideal hypnotic would be used long

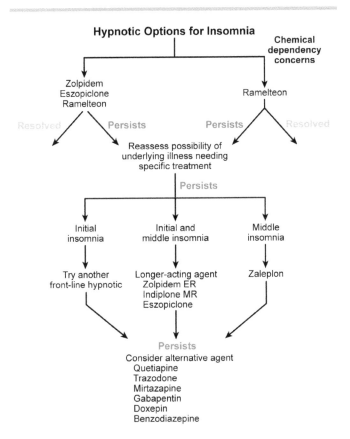

Figure 24 Hypnotic Options for Insomnia. The property of the hypnotic medication should be matched to the needs of the patient.

term without tolerance developing to its sedative qualities and without withdrawal on discontinuation.

Contemporary Hypnotics

The U.S. Food and Drug Administration has approved several benzodiazepines to treat primary insomnia, including flurazepam hydrochloride, triazolam, quazepam, estazolam, and temazepam. Benzodiazepines increase total sleep time with decreased initial sleep latency and reduced wakefulness after sleep onset. Of this group of medications, temazepam is particularly useful because of its intermediate-duration half-life and its lack of an active metabolite. When a clinician prefers to prescribe a benzodiazepine for insomnia, temazepam is a reasonable first choice (Table 10).

Agents other than benzodiazepines are increasingly used as the first-line treatment for insomnia (Table 11). Initially, the agents zaleplon and zolpidem tartrate were approved only for short-term treatment of insomnia. Most patients with insomnia who seek medical intervention have chronic symptoms, which creates an unfortunate mismatch of short-term treatment with a long-standing disorder. The 2005 National Institutes of Health Consensus Conference called for more clinical trials of treatments for chronic insomnia (16). Medications such as eszopiclone, zolpidem CR (extended release), and ramelteon have been approved for treatment of chronic insomnia without restrictions on longer-term use.

The benzodiazepine-receptor agonists do not share the chemical structure of benzodiazepines but do act on the benzodiazepine receptor interacting with the $GABA_A$ α_1 subunit that opens chloride channels (Figure 25). The benzodiazepine-receptor agonists are intended to be more selective than conventional benzodiazepines and thus cause less rebound insomnia and have a lower risk of being abused or contributing to respiratory depression. All the benzodiazepine-receptor agonists have a relatively short half-life that minimizes excessive daytime sleepiness and does not substantially alter sleep architecture.

Zolpidem is a selective agonist at the $GABA_A$ α_1 subunit that is preferentially found in the cortex. Because of its short half-life, this agent is used primarily to treat sleep-onset insomnia. The newer formulation of zolpidem CR has a biphasic release of the compound that facilitates the drug's ability to target both sleep onset and sleep maintenance insomnia (17). Zaleplon acts on a similar site and has a shorter half-life of about an hour. Like zolpidem, it is used primarily for sleep initiation or it can be used partway through the night to help patients with middle insomnia because of its long half-life. Eszopiclone is the S-isomer of the older medication zopiclone, used extensively outside the United States. On the basis of a six-month study (18), this medication was the first insomnia treatment approved for longer-term use. Eszopiclone is not associated with clinically significant tolerance or morning sedation. Sleep is improved with respect to decreased sleep latency, increased sleep efficiency, and increased total sleep time. However, patients using this medication have reported that it has an unpleasant taste (19). Like zolpidem, zaleplon and eszopiclone do not appear to alter normal sleep architecture.

The most novel pharmacologic agent for treatment of insomnia is ramelteon, which acts as an agonist on melatonin receptor types 1 and 2 (20). This agent has a different mechanism than that of the other GABAergic hypnotic agents. It is the only prescription hypnotic not classified by the U.S. Drug Enforcement Administration as a controlled substance. It has shown benefit for improving insomnia but its role with respect to circadian rhythm issues remains unclear.

Over the years, various agents not officially classified as hypnotics have been used as sleep aids. Clinicians may view antidepressants as a convenient way of addressing both insomnia and a coexisting mood disorder. The preferred agents have been mirtazapine, trazodone hydrochloride, and the tricyclic antidepressants. Unfortunately, these agents have not been carefully studied with respect to their sleep benefit. In particular, the duration of sedation may be excessive, leading to a hangover effect. They also may have multiple adverse effects, such as weight gain. Likewise, antipsychotic medications, particularly quetiapine fumarate, can sometimes be helpful. Atypical antipsychotic agents have been found to be especially helpful for patients with serious psychiatric disorders such as bipolar disorder, schizophrenia, or dementia with psychosis. However, in the absence of coexisting psychiatric disorders, the adverse effects of these medications should be carefully weighed against the benefits. For example, patients may be affected by weight gain and excessive daytime sleepiness.

Anticonvulsants have been used for various sleep complaints. Clonazepam is a benzodiazepine that is classified by the U.S. Food and Drug Administration as an anticonvulsant. Despite its long half-life, clonazepam can be helpful for patients who have difficulty sleeping, especially when their insomnia coexists with a parasomnia such as rapid eye movement (REM)

Table 10 Medication options for insomnia[a]

| Pharmacologic agent | | Drug class | Duration of action, h | Indications | Concerns |
Generic name	U.S. Trade name				
Temazepam[b]	Euhypnos, Norkotral, Normison, Remestan, Restoril, and Tenox	Benzodiazepine	8–15	Benzodiazepine-dependent insomnia; insomnia with existing RBD; insomnia with treatment-refractory RLS	Falls; cognitive impairment
Clonazepam	Klonopin	Benzodiazepine	8–15	Benzodiazepine-dependent insomnia; insomnia with existing RBD; insomnia with treatment-refractory RLS	Falls; cognitive impairment
Trazodone HCl	Desyrel, Molipaxin, Thombran, Trazorel, Trialodine, and Trittico	Antidepressant	8	Need to minimize chemical dependence risk	Falls; orthostatic hypotension; priapism
Mirtazapine	Remeron	Antidepressant	20–40	Insomnia in context of depression; minimize risk of addiction	Weight gain; less sedating at doses >15 mg
Doxepin	Adapin, Sinequan, and Zonalon	Antidepressant	8–24	Insomnia in context of depression or chronic pain	Constipation; dry mouth; orthostatic hypotension; cardiac conduction delay
Quetiapine fumarate	Ketipinor and Seroquel	Atypical antipsychotic	6	Insomnia in context of bipolar disorder or psychotic disorder; parasomnia (especially RBD in context of dementia with Lewy bodies); minimize CD risk	Weight gain; metabolic syndrome; slightly increased risk of stroke in dementia patients
Gabapentin	Neurontin	Anticonvulsant	5–7	Insomnia in context of RLS or chronic pain; hot flashes; minimizes CD risk; coexisting seizures	Unsteady gait at higher doses; poor clearance in patients with renal impairment

Abbreviations: CD, chemical dependency; HCl, hydrochloride; RBD, rapid eye-movement (REM) sleep behavior disorder; RLS, restless legs syndrome.
[a]Temazepam as a representative benzodiazepine plus other agents not classified as hypnotics.
[b]Approved for insomnia by the U.S. Food and Drug Administration.

Table 11 Hypnotic medications other than benzodiazepines

Pharmacologic agent		Initiates sleep	Maintains sleep	Appropriate for limited time in bed	Minimal required sleep time, h
Generic name	U.S. Trade name				
Eszopiclone	Lunesta	X	X		8
Ramelteon	Rozerem	X			2–5
Zaleplon	Sonata, Starnoc	X		X	4
Zolpidem tartrate	Ambien	X	X		7–8
Zolpidem tartrate CR	Ambien CR	X	X		7–8

Abbreviation: CR, extended release.

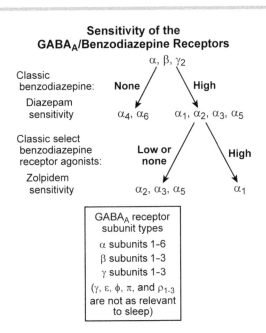

Figure 25 Sensitivity of the GABA$_A$/Benzodiazepine Receptors.

sleep behavior disorder. However, the long half-life also can lead to excessive daytime sleepiness. Some patients opt to obtain over-the-counter sleeping medications that contain diphenhydramine. These agents are widely used because they are available without a prescription. However, tolerance quickly develops, and the usefulness of these agents is considerably limited as a result. Lastly, antihistamines can contribute to cognitive impairment (21).

The variety and availability of hypnotics threaten to eclipse the role of behavioral therapies for insomnia. Several studies indicate that behavioral techniques offer more promise for sustained benefit. One response is to compromise by combining behavioral therapies with medications. This approach is optimal, especially when using behavioral therapy in isolation is not an option either due to the time lag in symptom improvement or the patient's lack of access to therapists. Relatively few studies have examined the value of combining these two approaches. Whether a patient may be as motivated to pursue behavioral therapy when medications

are concurrently prescribed has been a matter of debate (22). Nonetheless, in clinical practice this approach is commonplace. Patients often welcome the symptom relief they obtain from hypnotics. Ideally, patients can also be persuaded to look at their behaviors and attitudes that may have led to the development of insomnia or that may have perpetuated this condition.

REFERENCES

1. American Academy of Sleep Medicine. The International Classification of Sleep Disorders: Diagnostic and Coding Manual. 2nd ed. Westchester (IL): American Academy of Sleep Medicine, 2005.
2. Spielman AJ. Assessment of insomnia. Clin Psych Rev 1986; 6:11–25.
3. Nofzinger EA, Buysse DJ, Germain A, Price JC, Miewald JM, Kupfer DJ. Functional neuroimaging evidence for hyperarousal in insomnia. Am J Psychiatry 2004; 161:2126–8.
4. Perlis ML, Smith MT, Pigeon WR. Etiology and Pathophysiology of Insomnia. In: Kryger MH, Roth T, Dement WC, editors. Principles and Practice of Sleep Medicine. Philadelphia (PA): Elsevier Saunders, 2005. p. 714–25.
5. Dauvilliers Y, Morin C, Cervena K, et al. Family studies in insomnia. J Psychosom Res 2005; 58: 271–8.
6. Hamet P, Tremblay J. Genetics of the sleep-wake cycle and its disorders. Metabolism. 2006 (10 Suppl 1); S7–12.
7. Juang KD, Wang SJ, Lu SR, Lee SJ, Fuh JL. Hot flashes are associated with psychological symptoms of anxiety and depression in peri- and post- but not premenopausal women. Maturitas 2005; 52:119–26.
8. National Sleep Foundation Website [Internet] [cited 2009 Nov 10]. Available from http://www.sleepfoundation.org/.
9. Littner M, Hirshkowitz M, Kramer M, et al; American Academy of Sleep Medicine, Standards of Practice Committee. Practice parameters for using polysomnography to evaluate insomnia: an update. Sleep 2003; 26:754–60.
10. Salin-Pascual RJ, Roehrs TA, Merlotti LA, Zorick F, Roth T. Long-term study of the sleep of insomnia patients with sleep state misperception and other insomnia patients. Am J Psychiatry 1992; 149:904–8.
11. Hauri PJ. Sleep Hygiene, Relaxation Therapy, and Cognitive Interventions. In: Hauri PJ, editor. Case Studies in Insomnia. New York: Plenum Medical Book, 1991. p. 65–84.
12. Morin CM, Culbert JP, Schwartz SM. Nonpharmacological interventions for insomnia: a meta-analysis of treatment efficacy. Am J Psychiatry 1994; 151:1172–80.
13. Morgenthaler T, Kramer M, Alessi C, et al; American Academy of Sleep Medicine. Practice parameters for the psychological and behavioral treatment of insomnia: an update: an American Academy of Sleep Medicine report. Sleep 2006; 29:1415–9.
14. Smith MT, Huang MI, Manber R. Cognitive behavior therapy for chronic insomnia occurring within the context of medical and psychiatric disorders. Clin Psychol Rev 2005; 25:559–92.

15. Ritterband LM, Thorndike FP, Gonder-Frederick LA, et al. Efficacy of an Internet-based behavioral intervention for adults with insomnia. Arch Gen Psychiatry 2009; 66:692–8. Erratum in: Arch Gen Psychiatry 2010; 67: 311.

16. NIH State of the Science Conference statement on manifestations and management of chronic insomnia in adults statement. J Clin Sleep Med 2005; 1:412–21.

17. Scharf MB, Roth T, Vogel GW, Walsh JK. A multicenter, placebo-controlled study evaluating zolpidem in the treatment of chronic insomnia. J Clin Psychiatry 1994; 55:192–9.

18. Krystal AD, Walsh JK, Laska E, et al. Sustained efficacy of eszopiclone over 6 months of nightly treatment: results of a randomized, double-blind, placebo-controlled study in adults with chronic insominia. Sleep 2003; 26:793–9.

19. Zammit GK, Gillin JC, McNabb L, Caron J, Roth T. Eszopiclone, a novel non-benzodiazepine anti-insomnia agent: a six-week efficacy and safety study in adult patients with chronic insomnia [abstract]. Sleep 2003; 26(Suppl): A297.

20. Richardson GS, Zammit G, Wang-Weigand S, Zhang J. Safety and subjective sleep effects of ramelteon administration in adults and older adults with chronic primary insomnia: a 1-year, open-label study. J Clin Psychiatry 2009; 70:467–76. Epub 2009 Mar 10.

21. Witek TJ Jr, Canestrari DA, Miller RD, Yang JY, Riker DK. Characterization of daytime sleepiness and psychomotor performance following H1 receptor antagonists. Ann Allergy Asthma Immunol 1995; 74:419–26.

22. Hauri PJ. Can we mix behavioral therapy with hypnotics when treating insomniacs? Sleep 1997; 20:1111–8.

9

Movement Disorders and Parasomnias

Michael H. Silber, MBChB, FCP (SA)

ABBREVIATIONS

NREM, non–rapid eye movement

RBD, rapid eye movement sleep behavior disorder

REM, rapid eye movement

RLS, restless legs syndrome

Abnormal movements and sensory perceptions during the night are rather arbitrarily divided into sleep-related movement disorders and parasomnias (1). Nocturnal seizures are considered a separate category of disorder, although they are commonly considered in the differential diagnosis of the other conditions. Clinical acumen and experience are often needed to identify the correct diagnosis from this fascinating spectrum of disorders.

SLEEP-RELATED MOVEMENT DISORDERS
Restless Legs Syndrome

In 1945 Doctor Karl-Axel Ekbom of Sweden published a 123-page monograph entitled *Restless Legs* (Figure 1) (2). This seminal work, with its meticulous clinical descriptions, was the first clear presentation about what has proven to be one of the most common sleep disorders. About 5% to 10% of the population experiences restless legs syndrome (RLS) (3–5), with severity ranging from an intermittent mild annoyance to a devastating disorder causing profound insomnia, daytime fatigue, and intense distress.

RLS is characterized by four clinical criteria: 1) an irresistible urge to move the legs, usually but not always associated with discomfort; 2) occurrence at rest (while sitting or lying down); 3) at least temporary relief by movement; and 4) worsening of symptoms during the evening or at night (6). There are no tests with high sensitivity or specificity, and RLS is usually diagnosed on the basis of the patient's history. Periodic limb movements of sleep on polysomnography are found in about 85% of patients with RLS (7), but these movements are nonspecific, being associated with a range of other sleep disorders as well as occurring with high frequency in normal older persons (Figure 2) (8). Some patients with RLS describe spontaneous jerking of the legs at rest while awake, which is known as *periodic limb movements of wakefulness* (Figure 3). RLS is more common in women, and it can start at any age, including during childhood.

Current concepts of the pathogenesis of RLS center on a presumed dopamine deficiency in the basal ganglia that is associated with reduced iron content in regions of the brain. At least 50% of patients have a family history of the disorder, especially if the symptoms commence before 50 years of age (7). The usual inheritance pattern is autosomal dominant, and linkages have been found to six chromosomal sites (Table 1). Genome-wide association studies have also identified predisposing polymorphisms on several genes (Table 2), but a coherent picture of the genetic influences contributing to the disorder has not yet emerged. Systemic iron deficiency, caused by conditions such as menorrhagia, gastrointestinal blood loss, or frequent blood donation, have been clearly associated with RLS; more severe symptoms are linked to serum ferritin concentrations in the low normal to low range (<50 mcg/L) (18). Cerebrospinal ferritin concentrations are lower in RLS patients than in controls, even in the presence of normal serum ferritin levels (19), and magnetic resonance imaging and autopsy studies have revealed low iron content in the basal ganglia (Figure 4) (20). The mechanism underlying low cerebral iron stores and the relation between iron and dopamine deficiency require further elucidation. Other associations with RLS include chronic renal failure, peripheral neuropathy, pregnancy, and the use of antidepressants, antihistamines, and neuroleptic agents.

Management of RLS (Figure 5) commences with nonpharmacologic approaches (21). Physical activity, warm baths, massage, and mental alerting techniques can provide symptom relief. Some patients may benefit from a reduction in caffeine, nicotine, or alcohol intake. If low iron stores are detected, supplementation with oral iron preparations may be beneficial. Open-label studies of intravenous iron therapy have yielded promising results, but one controlled trial was stopped due to a lack of efficacy (22).

Four groups of medications have been found useful in RLS management, and most patients can be helped by drug therapy. Dopaminergic agents, especially nonergot agonists such as pramipexole and ropinirole, are the first-line drugs for daily treatment of RLS (23). Antiseizure medications, especially gabapentin, are useful alternative or additional agents, whereas benzodiazepines may assist in providing relief by enhancing sleep. The opioids are highly effective agents, with high-potency opioids having a distinct role to play in treating refractory disease.

The dopaminergic agents (especially levodopa) can induce a phenomenon known as *augmentation* (24), defined as an exacerbation of RLS that occurs after the commencement of treatment. It is usually characterized by the development of new RLS symptoms at a time of day before administration of the medication. Symptoms may also spread to the arms or increase in intensity. Augmentation occurs in 85% of patients taking levodopa and in about 32% of patients taking dopamine

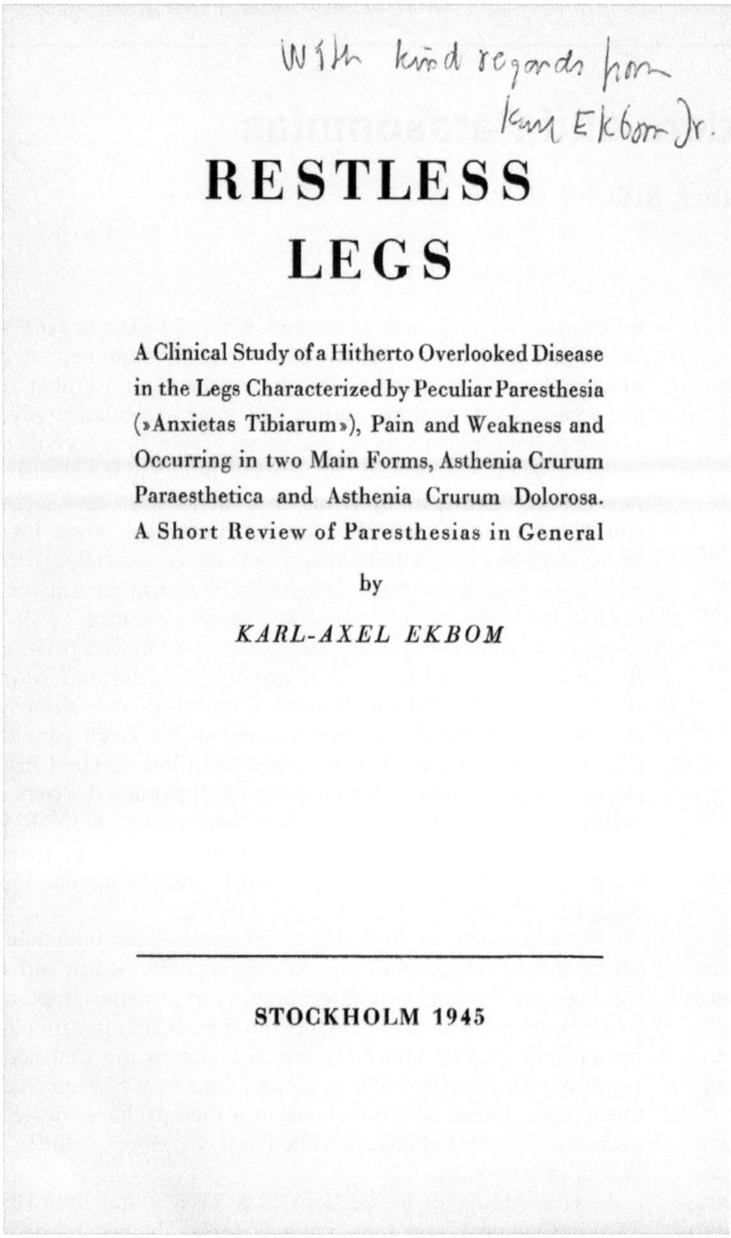

RESTLESS LEGS

A Clinical Study of a Hitherto Overlooked Disease in the Legs Characterized by Peculiar Paresthesia (»Anxietas Tibiarum»), Pain and Weakness and Occurring in two Main Forms, Asthenia Crurum Paraesthetica and Asthenia Crurum Dolorosa. A Short Review of Paresthesias in General

by

KARL-AXEL EKBOM

STOCKHOLM 1945

Figure 1 Cover Page of First Comprehensive Monograph on Restless Legs Syndrome. In 1945 Dr Karl-Axel Ekbom, a Swedish neurologist, published the first comprehensive account of a disorder he called *restless legs*. His 123-page monograph covers clinical features, differential diagnosis, etiology, and therapy. Although concepts about the pathogenesis of restless legs syndrome and its therapy have evolved since Ekbom's day, his description of the symptoms remains detailed, accurate, and vivid. (From Ekbom KA [2].)

agonists. The underlying mechanisms are poorly understood. Dopamine agonists can sometimes cause daytime sleepiness and impulse control disorders, such as compulsive gambling (25). The ergot agonists, such as cabergoline and pergolide, are seldom used today because of their tendency to cause cardiac valvular fibrosis.

Other Sleep-Related Movement Disorders

Periodic limb movement disorder consists of insomnia or hypersomnia in patients with periodic limb movements during sleep who do not have RLS or any other sleep disorder that can better explain their symptoms (1). As periodic limb movements are generally asymptomatic epiphenomena of other sleep disorders or of aging, considerable caution should be exercised in relating the movements observed on a polysomnogram to the clinical complaints. Treatment of periodic limb movement disorder is similar to that for RLS.

Sleep-related leg cramps are characterized by sudden painful spasms of leg muscles that wake the patient from sleep. In contrast to RLS, sleep-related cramps cause the muscle to feel hard upon palpation, and relief can best be obtained by massaging the cramp or standing on the leg rather than by walking. Most cases of sleep-related leg cramps are idiopathic. Treatment is difficult; quinine has been suggested, but controlled trials are unconvincing and quinine preparations have

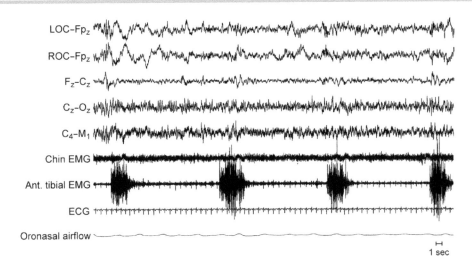

Figure 2 Periodic Limb Movements of Sleep. Periodic limb movements of sleep (PLMS) can be found in 85% of patients with restless legs syndrome but are nonspecific, often accompanying other sleep disorders such as obstructive sleep apnea and narcolepsy. This polysomnogram fragment shows PLMS. The duration of an individual movement is 0.5 to 10 seconds, the amplitude at least 8 microvolts, and the intermovement interval 5 to 90 seconds. At least 4 movements must occur successively in order for them to be classified as PLMS. Ant. tibial indicates anterior tibial muscles; ECG, electrocardiogram; EMG, electromyogram; LOC, left outer canthus; Oronasal airflow, airflow recorded by nasal pressure transducer; ROC, right outer canthus.

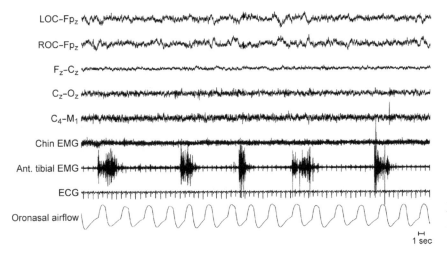

Figure 3 Periodic Limb Movements of Wakefulness. Periodic limb movements of wakefulness frequently accompany restless legs syndrome, as can be seen on this polysomnogram fragment. For explanation of labels, see Figure 2.

Table 1 Genetic linkage studies in restless legs syndrome

Genetic Subtypes	Population	Linkage	Inheritance	Reference
RLS 1	French Canadian	12q	Autosomal recessive	Desautels et al, 2001 (9)
RLS 2	Italian	14q	Autosomal dominant	Bonati et al, 2003 (10)
RLS 3	United States	9p	Autosomal dominant	Chen et al, 2004 (11)
RLS 4	French Canadian	20p	Autosomal dominant	Levchenko et al, 2006 (12)
RLS 5	Italian Tyrol	2q	Autosomal dominant	Pichler et al, 2006 (13)
RLS 6	Italian	19p	Autosomal dominant	Kemlink et al, 2008 (14)

Abbreviation: RLS, restless legs syndrome.

Table 2 Genome-wide association studies in restless legs syndrome

Population	Disorder	Chromosome	Gene	Protein	Reference
French Canadian; European	RLS	2p	MEIS-1	Expressed in substantia nigra; spinal motor neuron connectivity; limb formation	Winkelmann et al, 2007 (15)
French Canadian; European; Icelandic	RLS and PLMS	6p	BTBD9	Widely expressed in brain	Winkelmann et al, 2007 (15) Stefansson et al, 2007 (16)
French Canadian; European	RLS	15q	MAP2K5-LBOXCOR1	Neuroprotection of dopamine neurons; development of sensory pathways in spinal cord dorsal horn	Winkelmann et al, 2007 (15)
Icelandic; United States	PLMS	6p	GLO1	Glycoxalase 1 (glycolytic pathway)	Stefansson et al, 2007 (16)
Icelandic; United States	PLMS	6p	DNAH8	Microtubule-associated complex	Stefansson et al, 2007 (16)
European; Canadian	RLS	9p	PTPRD	Embryonic axon guidance of motor neurons	Schormair et al, 2008 (17)

Abbreviations: PLMS, periodic limb movements of sleep; RLS, restless legs syndrome.

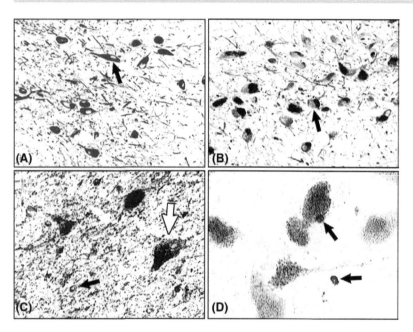

Figure 4 Reduced Iron Stores in the Brains of Patients With Restless Legs Syndrome. Seven brains from patients with restless legs syndrome were compared with the brains of 5 controls. The number of substantia nigra neuromelanin cells immunostaining for tyrosine hydroxylase was compared. (A and B) In both of these parts of Figure 4, neuromelanin stains brown and tyrosine hydroxylase stains blue. (Arrows point to typical cells as examples.) There was no significant difference between the brains of controls (A) and those of persons with restless legs syndrome (RLS) (B). (C and D) In both of these parts of Figure 4, the sections were stained for H-ferritin (blue). In the control brain (C), H-ferritin can be seen in the neuromelanin cells (white arrow) and in the parenchyma (black arrow). In contrast, in the RLS brain (D), there is no detectable H-ferritin in the neuromelanin cells and H-ferritin is present in only a few glial cells (black arrows). These findings are consistent with absent iron stores in the substantia nigra neurons in RLS brains. (From Connor JR, Boyer PJ, Menzies SL, et al. Neuropathological examination suggests impaired brain iron acquisition in restless legs syndrome. Neurology 2003; 61:304–9. [Used with permission.])

the potential for serious cardiac and hematologic side effects (26). The only quinine preparation still being marketed in the United States is not approved for the treatment of leg cramps.

Sleep-related rhythmic movement disorder is characterized by regular stereotyped contractions of large muscle groups that occur during drowsiness or sleep (Figure 6) (1). It includes body rocking and head banging, but it may occasionally manifest as other movements such as leg jerking. Rhythmic movement disorder falls into a twilight area between involuntary movements and quasi-voluntary activity. Many patients report being aware of their movements when they are lying in bed and indicate that they have always moved their body to facilitate the onset of sleep. However, the movements often persist into

stage N1 and stage N2 sleep and occasionally can even be observed during rapid eye movement (REM) sleep. Rhythmic movement disorder is extremely common in infants but usually resolves by five years of age. However, in some patients it may persist into adulthood. It is more common in mentally handicapped or autistic children, who might have to wear a helmet to protect the head from injury. Drug therapy is rarely helpful.

Sleep-related bruxism is a common complaint (27,28) that consists of grinding the teeth during sleep (Figure 7). Bruxism may result in jaw pain and physical damage to the teeth. It is most common during stage N1 and stage N2 sleep, and it can sometimes be seen during arousal from episodes of sleep apnea. Treatment usually involves the wearing of a dental protection device at night.

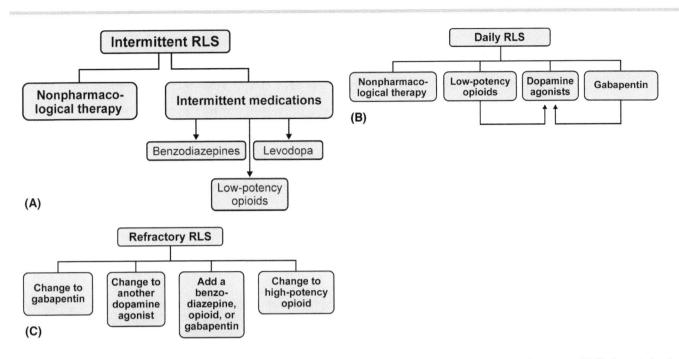

(A)

(B)

(C)

Figure 5 Management of Restless Legs Syndrome. The Medical Advisory Board of the Restless Legs Syndrome (RLS) Foundation has formulated an algorithm for the management of RLS. (A) Intermittent RLS is troublesome enough to require treatment but does not occur sufficiently often to require daily therapy. (B) Daily RLS is troublesome and occurs frequently enough to require daily therapy. (C) Refractory RLS has been treated with a dopamine agonist, resulting in at least one of the following outcomes: inadequate response, intolerable side effects, development of tolerance, or uncontrollable daytime augmentation. (From Silber MH, Ehrenberg BL, Allen RP, et al; Medical Advisory Board of the Restless Legs Syndrome Foundation. An algorithm for the management of restless legs syndrome. Mayo Clin Proc 2004; 79: 916-22. [Used with permission.])

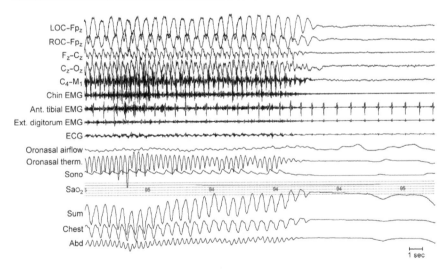

Figure 6 Rhythmic Movement Disorder. This 30-second polysomnogram fragment shows movement artifact at 1.5 Hz visible on the electro-oculogram, electroencephalogram, and respiratory channels. The patient rocked his head from side to side at the same frequency. Abd indicates abdominal inductance plethysmography; Chest, thoracic inductance plethysmography; Ext. digitorum, extensor digitorum communis; Oronasal therm., oronasal thermocouple; Sao$_2$, arterial oxygen saturation; Sono, recording of upper airway sound; Sum, the arithmetic sum of the signals of chest and abdominal inductance plethysmography. For explanation of other labels, see Figure 2.

PARASOMNIAS

Parasomnias are undesirable, paroxysmal, motor, or sensory phenomena that occur during sleep. Parasomnias are classified according to the state of sleep from which they arise: non–rapid eye movement (NREM) parasomnias, REM parasomnias, or non–state-dependent parasomnias. Many of the terrifying nighttime phenomena of folklore, such as incubi and night hags, are due to parasomnias.

The diagnosis of a parasomnia can often be made by taking a careful history from the patient and bed partner or another observer, especially when the disorder manifests in childhood. However, when the diagnosis is uncertain, further

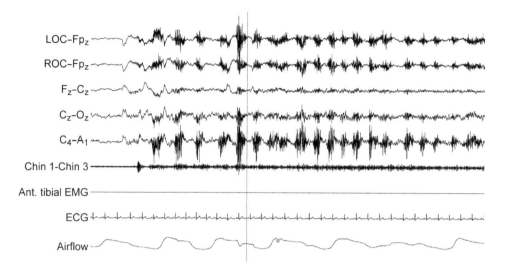

Figure 7 Bruxism. This 30-second polysomnogram fragment indicates rhythmic electromyogram activity from the outer canthi and mastoid electrodes at a frequency of 0.5 to 1 Hz. These findings are typical of bruxism. Airflow indicates oronasal airflow recorded by nasal pressure transducer. For explanation of other labels, see Figure 2.

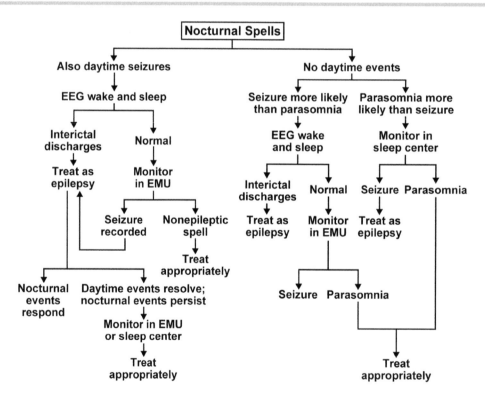

Figure 8 Diagnostic Approach to Events Occurring During Sleep. This algorithm offers a diagnostic approach to interpreting events that occur during sleep when there is doubt about whether the diagnosis is a parasomnia or a seizure disorder. EEG indicates electroencephalogram; EMU, epilepsy monitoring unit. (From Silber MH, Krahn LE, Morgenthaler TI. Sleep Medicine in Clinical Practice. New York: Taylor & Francis, 2004. [Used with permission of Mayo Foundation for Medical Education and Research.])

studies are required, especially if either a seizure disorder or obstructive sleep apnea are possible alternatives or if the events are potentially injurious to the patient or others (Figure 8). Although a wake and sleep electroencephalogram and mag-

netic resonance imaging scan of the brain may be important for some patients, the most useful investigation is extended polysomnography. Video electroencephalographic polysomnography consists of a traditional comprehensive polysomnogram

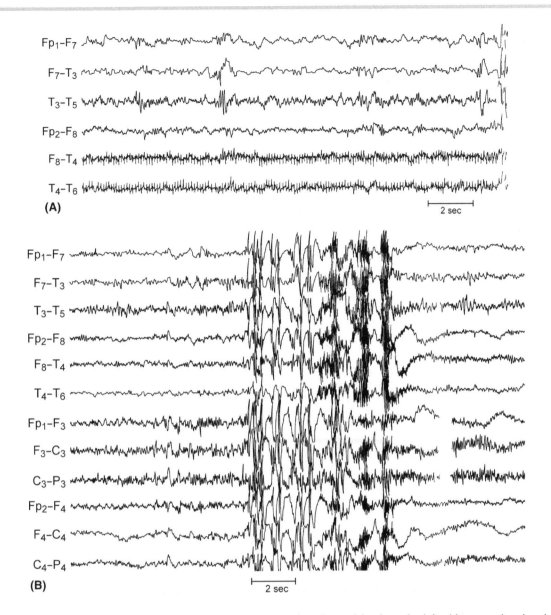

Figure 9 Epileptiform Activity During Sleep. (A) Potentially epileptogenic spikes arising from the left mid-temporal region during non–rapid eye movement (NREM) sleep are apparent on this fragment of an electroencephalogram (EEG) recording, which was obtained during a polysomnogram with additional EEG derivations. This interictal activity is a marker of predisposition to partial seizures. (B) Generalized epileptiform spike and wave activity arousing the patient from NREM sleep. (From Silber MH, Krahn LE, Morgenthaler TI. Sleep Medicine in Clinical Practice. New York: Taylor & Francis, 2004. [Used with permission of Mayo Foundation for Medical Education and Research.])

combined with an additional 16 electroencephalographic derivations, additional arm surface electromyography, and time-synchronized video and audio recordings (29). Interpreters of these studies should be familiar with the polysomnographic manifestations of sleep-disordered breathing as well as with the electroencephalographic changes caused by seizures (Figure 9). The primary goal, of course, is to record one of the patient's typical events. However, even if such a recording cannot be obtained, helpful information may be gleaned from a careful review of the record: increased muscle tone during REM sleep suggests REM sleep behavior disorder (RBD); the presence of confusional arousals suggests that sleepwalking may occur on other nights; and interictal spike discharges may be evidence of a seizure disorder.

Parasomnias Associated With NREM Sleep

The arousal disorders are characterized by abnormal behavior following sudden partial arousals from NREM, usually slow-wave sleep (Figure 10) (30). These disorders include sleepwalking, sleep terrors, and confusional arousals, but the clinical manifestations often overlap among the three entities. Events occur generally in the first third of the night, corresponding to the timing of most slow-wave sleep. Patients are unresponsive to external stimuli during the arousal events and are usually confused when awakened, with little memory of what transpired. Dream recall is rare. In classic sleepwalking, the patient exhibits coordinated motor activity, such as standing by the bed or walking around. Sleep terrors manifest with autonomic, motor, and vocal manifestations of intense fear, whereas

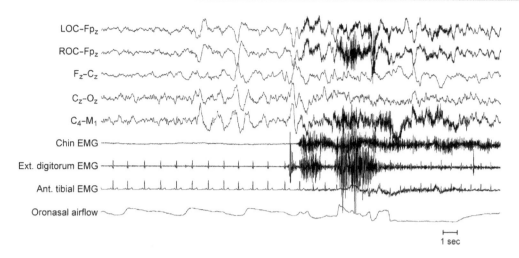

Figure 10 Confusional Arousal. A 30-second polysomnogram shows a sudden arousal from slow-wave sleep followed by muscle artifact and mixed-frequency electroencephalographic (EEG) activity. The patient sat up and fidgeted with the EEG leads. Ext. digitorum indicates extensor digitorum communis. For explanation of other labels, see Figure 2.

patients with confusional arousals generally appear disorientated but have neither the complex mobility of sleepwalking nor the severe fright of sleep terrors. Arousal disorders are common in childhood, and as many as 2% to 4% of adults report walking in their sleep (31,32).

The pathophysiology of arousal disorders remains obscure. Patients appear to be "entrapped" between the states of slow-wave sleep and wakefulness, with possibly a blunted arousal response. The high frequency of arousal disorders in young persons suggests the possibility of delayed maturation of the neural pathways that mediate the transition to wake, possibly with a genetic basis, as evidenced by the occurrence of many familial cases. Numerous factors precipitate the events on any particular night. These include circumstances that deepen slow-wave sleep, such as rebound from sleep deprivation or unusual sleep-wake cycles, medications that prevent complete awakening from sleep, and factors that increase arousals, such as environmental noise, medical conditions including sleep apnea, and psychological stress (Figure 11).

Violent behavior during arousal parasomnias is rare but can have profound consequences (33). Sleepwalkers have been known to throw themselves out of windows, sometimes resulting in severe injuries. Sleepwalkers may walk into furniture, leave their homes, and very occasionally even start up and drive their cars. Violence against others rarely occurs, but there have been documented cases of physical and sexual assault or even homicide perpetrated by sleepwalkers. To successfully sustain a claim that such behaviors occurred while asleep, the assailant must provide evidence of a past history of sleepwalking, should have had no motive for the assault, should react with perplexity and horror to being told about it, and should have made no attempt at concealment when confronted with the consequences of the actions (34).

Management of noninjurious parasomnias in children may often only involve reassurance to the parents that the events are of little clinical consequence and that most children will outgrow them. Treatment may be needed if the events are violent or dangerous, disruptive to the family, or result in

embarrassment, such as while away from home (e.g., during sleepovers or while away at college). Behavioral techniques include addressing sleep hygiene, hypnosis (35), or scheduled anticipatory awakenings in which the patient is awakened a few minutes before the habitual time of the events. Medications that may be effective include the intermediate- or long-acting benzodiazepines, such as clonazepam (36). Short-acting hypnotics, such as zolpidem, should be used with caution, as they may sometimes induce sleepwalking themselves (37).

Parasomnias Associated With REM Sleep
RBD is characterized by loss of the skeletal muscle atonia that characterizes normal REM sleep and resultant complex motor activity associated with dreaming (38,39). For unknown reasons, about 90% of patients with RBD are men. It is predominantly a disorder of middle to older age, with the mean age of onset being reported in different series as 53 and 61 years. However, RBD has been identified in younger patients, including children. Patients kick, flail their arms, punch, shout, and scream during REM sleep. These behaviors can be injurious to the patients and their bed partners: patients may throw themselves out of bed, sometimes causing severe personal injuries, and they may punch, slap, kick, or even throttle their bed partners. Dreams may change and become more violent; usually patients with RBD dream that they are being attacked by a person or an animal and are trying to defend themselves when they inadvertently assault their bed partners. There is no change in their waking personality; however, one study showed that RBD patients scored lower than controls on daytime aggression scales (40). The polysomnogram shows increased muscle tone during the REM sleep of persons with RBD (Figure 12). Even if actual events are not recorded in the laboratory, the loss of REM sleep atonia and the presence of a typical history are diagnostic of the disorder.

RBD is closely related to neurodegenerative disorders, especially the synucleinopathies, which include Parkinson disease, dementia with Lewy bodies, and multiple system atrophy (41).

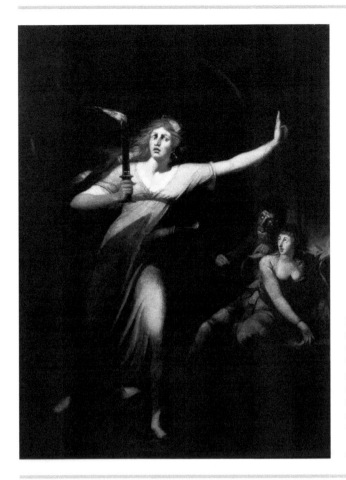

Figure 11 Lady Macbeth Sleepwalking. Lady Macbeth, a central character in William Shakespeare's play, *Macbeth,* is perhaps the most famous fictional sleepwalker. Tormented by the murder of King Duncan, which she and her husband planned and he executed, she walks in her sleep, trying to wash off the blood she imagines is on her hands. Shakespeare's dialogue shows that he understood the essence of sleepwalking. The watching doctor comments, "You see, her eyes are open," to which Lady Macbeth's gentlewoman in waiting replies, "Ay, but their sense is shut." (Act V, Scene 1, *Macbeth.*) (Oil on canvas titled *Lady Macbeth Sleep Walking* [1784] by John Henry Fuseli.) (From the Musée du Louvre, Paris, France. [Used with permission.])

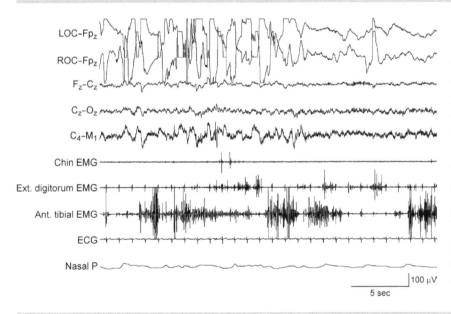

Figure 12 Rapid Eye Movement Sleep Behavior Disorder. This fragment of a polysomnogram shows abnormally increased electromyographic (EMG) activity during rapid eye movement sleep. This activity is especially noticeable in the limb muscle derivations, which emphasizes the importance of recording more than just the chin EMG. This patient presented with dream enactment behavior, including shouting, punching, and kicking during the night, and he later recalled dreaming about defending himself against attack. (From Silber MH, Krahn LE, Morgenthaler TI. Sleep Medicine in Clinical Practice. New York: Taylor & Francis, 2004. [Used with permission of Mayo Foundation for Medical Education and Research.]) Ext. digitorum indicates extensor digitorum communis; Nasal P, nasal pressure. For explanation of other labels, see Figure 2.

It has been detected in 15% to 33% of patients with Parkinson disease (42) and in 60% to 90% of patients with multiple system atrophy (43,44). There is extensive convergent evidence that Lewy body disease will develop in most patients with idiopathic RBD, and thus RBD alone most often represents an early manifestation of this disorder. Of 29 patients with idiopathic RBD in one study, Parkinsonism or dementia developed in 65%, a mean of 13 years after onset of RBD (45). Autopsy findings of extensive Lewy

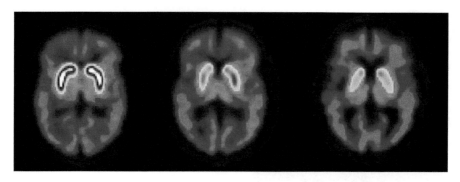

Figure 13 Positron Emission Tomography Studies Show Rapid Eye Movement Sleep Behavior Disorder as a Precursor of Parkinson Disease. Six patients with rapid eye movement sleep behavior disorder (RBD) without definite Parkinsonism and 19 age-matched control subjects underwent positron emission tomography scans performed with [^{11}C]dihydrotetrabenazine (DTBZ). DTBZ binds to the brain vesicular monoamine transporter, and its density in the striatum is a measure of the number of dopaminergic neurons in the substantia nigra. Significant reduction in DTBZ binding was found in the striatum of two of the patients (middle and right) compared with that of the controls (left). This finding suggests that patients with RBD have reduced dopaminergic neurons in the substantia nigra, which is compatible with subclinical Parkinson disease. RBD is often an early marker of Lewy bodies pathology. (From Albin RL, Koeppe RA, Chervin RD, et al. Decreased striatal dopaminergic innervation in REM sleep behavior disorder. Neurology 2000; 55:1410-12. [Used with permission.])

bodies were reported in two RBD patients with normal neurological examinations at the time of death (41,46). Otherwise asymptomatic RBD patients have been shown to exhibit subtle changes in visuospatial function, olfaction, autonomic function, electroencephalographic power, and positron emission tomography (Figure 13) (47). Not all RBD patients have a neurodegenerative disorder. RBD can occur with antidepressant treatment, narcolepsy, and, rarely, with structural lesions affecting the lower brainstem (Figures 14-16) (41,48). Management includes improving the safety of the bedroom environment by moving furniture away from the bed and sometimes placing cushions or a soft mattress on the floor adjacent to the bed. The most effective medication is clonazepam, with about a 90% success rate in open-label studies (38,39). Unfortunately,

this drug can cause sleepiness, cognitive impairment, gait unsteadiness, and impotence in older patients, especially in those with a neurodegenerative disorder. An alternative agent is melatonin, which has been found to be effective in several open-label studies (49-51).

Nightmare disorder is characterized by recurrent frightening dreams. Although occasional nightmares are common and of little clinical significance, recurrent nightmares should raise suspicion of posttraumatic stress disorder. Nightmares differ from sleep terrors in that they arise from REM sleep and are associated with vivid dream recall, and they differ from RBD by the absence of motor activity. *Recurrent isolated sleep paralysis* consists of repeated episodes of paralysis of voluntary muscles, accompanied by the inability to speak or move the

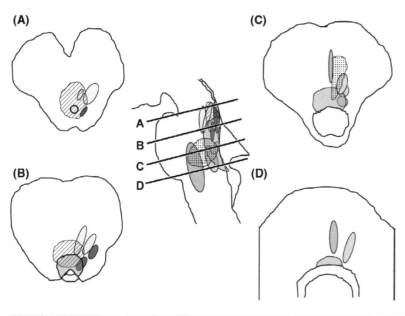

Figure 14 Association of Lesions Causing Rapid Eye Movement Sleep Behavior Disorder With Brainstem Neurons. This schematic figure shows the overlap between lesions reported to cause rapid eye movement sleep behavior disorder (RBD) and areas of the brainstem known to be associated with rapid eye movement (REM) sleep. The red areas represent the REM-off regions and the green areas represent the REM-on regions. The orange area is the raphe nuclei, the blue area is the locus coeruleus and the yellow regions are the lateral dorsal tegmental and pedunculopontine nuclei. The gray and hatched regions indicate lesions in three patients with RBD due to multiple sclerosis, a cavernous hemangioma, or an infarct. As can be seen, there is considerable overlap of the lesions with the neuronal groups associated with REM sleep. Figures A to D show transverse sections through the brainstem at the levels indicated on the midline sagittal section. (From Boeve BF, Silber MH, Saper CB, et al. Pathophysiology of REM sleep behaviour disorder and relevance to neurodegenerative disease. Brain 2007; 130:2770-88. [Used with permission.])

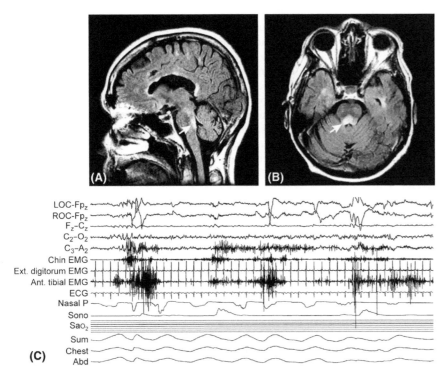

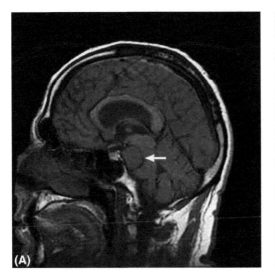

Figure 15 A Case of Rapid Eye Movement Sleep Behavior Disorder and Multiple Sclerosis. A 51-year-old woman with known multiple sclerosis had an acute attack of rapid eye movement sleep behavior disorder that affected the brainstem and was accompanied by vertigo, dysarthria, ataxia, diplopia, and bifacial weakness. She had an acute onset of dream enactment behavior, with screaming, groaning, flailing, and thrashing. T2-weighted magnetic resonance imaging ([A] midline sagittal view and [B] transverse view) showed an area of inflammation in the dorsal pons (A and B [arrow]), whereas polysomnography (C) showed increased muscle tone during REM sleep. Abd indicates abdominal plethysmography; Chest, rib cage plethysmography; Ext. digitorum, extensor digitorum communis; Nasal P, nasal pressure; Sao$_2$, arterial oxygen saturation; Sono, recording of upper airway sound; Sum, the arithmetic sum of rib cage and abdominal plethysmography. For explanation of other labels, see Figure 2. (From Tippmann-Peikert M, Boeve BF, Keegan BM. REM sleep behavior disorder initiated by acute brainstem multiple sclerosis. Neurology 2006; 66:1277-9. [Used with permission.])

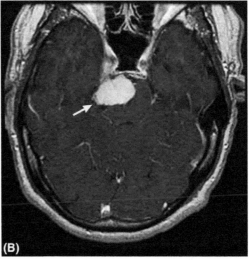

Figure 16 An Extra-Axial Brain Tumor Causing Rapid Eye Movement Sleep Behavior Disorder. A 64-year-old man presented with a two-year history of daily dream-enactment behavior due to rapid eye movement sleep behavior disorder (RBD). He would flail his arms, yell, kick, and hit the wall or his wife. He dreamed that he was being chased by animals. For the preceding nine months before presentation, he had noticed diplopia, decreased cognition, and shuffling gait. Examination revealed a right abducens neuropathy and a left hemiparesis. Magnetic resonance imaging showed a large right clivus meningioma (A and B [arrows]) compressing and displacing the pons and causing hydrocephalus. (A) T1-weighted sagittal view without contrast; (B) T1-weighted axial view with contrast. After the hydrocephalus was shunted and the meningioma was resected, the patient had complete resolution of the dream-enactment behavior.

limbs at sleep onset or upon awakening in the absence of narcolepsy. These events appear to arise from REM sleep and may be associated with hallucinatory experiences. They generally commence during adolescence and resolve later in life without clinical consequences.

Non–State-Dependent Parasomnias

Sleep-related eating disorder is a parasomnia in which patients, most commonly women, leave their beds to eat but later have little or no recall of their actions (52). Patients often eat unusual combinations of high-calorie food in a sloppy manner. Sleep-related eating disorder has been associated with other forms of sleepwalking, affective disorders, anxiety disorder, prior substance abuse, sleep apnea, and RLS. It can occur in patients taking short-acting hypnotics, especially zolpidem (37). The differential diagnosis includes night-eating syndrome in which patients, with full awareness, consume more than half their daily caloric intake during the night and then have early morning satiety. These two conditions may be related because some patients show variable recall of their night eating (53). In addition, the use of zolpidem has been known to transform voluntary night eating into amnestic sleep eating. Treatment of sleep-related eating disorder is challenging. Comorbid conditions, including sleep apnea and RLS, should be treated, and short-acting hypnotics should be discontinued. Longer-acting agents such as temazepam or clonazepam may be helpful. Topiramate has been suggested as a possible therapeutic agent (54).

Sleep-related groaning (catathrenia) is a rare phenomenon characterized by deep inspirations followed by prolonged expirations during which the patient makes a monotonous groaning sound (Figure 17) (55,56). The events occur predominantly during REM sleep but the sleeper's muscles remain atonic. The only apparent consequence is disruption of the sleep of the bed partner. The disorder usually commences in early adulthood and is more common in men. Its pathophysiology is unknown. Management is extremely difficult, but some cases respond to continuous positive airway pressure.

Sleep-related hallucinations include multimodal hallucinatory experiences at sleep onset (hypnagogic hallucinations), as well as complex visual hallucinations on waking during the night. Although hypnagogic hallucinations may be associated with narcolepsy, in isolation they are extremely common and are not considered pathologic. Complex nocturnal hallucinations, which are characterized by vivid figures of distorted people and animals, occur after waking during sleep and usually last less than 5 minutes, disappearing when a light is switched on (57). They may be associated with a number of different etiologies, including anxiety disorder, the use of β-adrenergic antagonists, Lewy body disease, and visual loss (Charles Bonnet syndrome [release hallucinations]).

Exploding head syndrome is characterized by an impression of a usually painless explosion in the head or a sudden loud noise that occurs at the transition between wake and sleep or sleep and wake (1). Its pathophysiology is unknown, but the condition appears to be a sensory analogue of the more

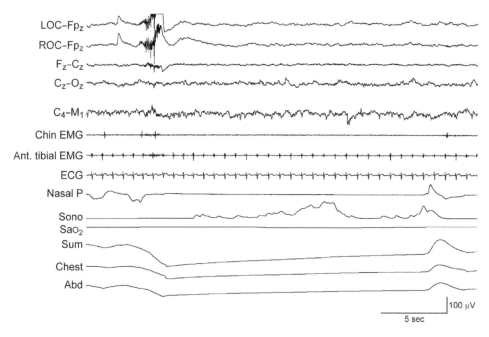

Figure 17 Sleep-Related Groaning (Catathrenia). This 30-second polysomnogram fragment shows catathrenia (prolonged expiratory groaning) during rapid eye movement sleep. Expiration is indicated by upward deflections in the airflow and impedance of plethysmography channels. On these two channels, note the 20-second prolonged expiration with slowly rising signals commencing at the end of an inspiratory breath. The sonogram channel demonstrates accompanying vocalization during expiration, which on an audio recording would sound like a prolonged moan. Abd indicates abdominal plethysmography; Chest, rib cage plethysmography; Nasal P, nasal pressure; Sono, recording of upper airway sound; Sao₂, arterial oxygen saturation; Sum, the arithmetic sum of rib cage and abdominal plethysmography. For explanation of other labels, see Figure 2. (From Silber MH, Krahn LE, Morgenthaler TI. Sleep Medicine in Clinical Practice. New York: Taylor & Francis, 2004. [Used with permission of Mayo Foundation for Medical Education and Research.])

common benign sleep starts, which manifest as sudden jerks of the body at sleep onset.

Sleep-related dissociative disorders are psychogenic dissociative events that occur during wakefulness after arousal from sleep. Most patients with this disorder also manifest dissociative behaviors during the day. It is important to differentiate this entity from the arousal parasomnias.

Sleep enuresis consists of the involuntary voiding of urine after an age (about 5 years) at which a child can generally maintain bladder control throughout the night. Urologic abnormalities should be excluded. Management involves the use of behavioral techniques and occasionally the administration of nasal desmopressin.

REFERENCES

1. American Academy of Sleep Medicine. The International Classification of Sleep Disorders: Diagnostic and Coding Manual. 2nd ed. Westchester (IL): American Academy of Sleep Medicine, 2005.
2. Ekbom KA. Restless Legs: A Clinical Study of a Hitherto Overlooked Disease in the Legs Characterized by Peculiar Paresthesia ("Anxietas Tibiarum"), Pain and Weakness and Occurring in Two Main Forms, Asthenia Crurum Paraesthetica and Asthenia Crurum Dolorosa: A Short Review of Paresthesias in General. Stockholm: Ivar Hoeggstroms, 1945.
3. Hogl B, Kiechl S, Willeit J, et al. Restless legs syndrome: a community-based study of prevalence, severity, and risk factors. Neurology 2005; 64:1920–4.
4. Nichols DA, Allen RP, Grauke JH, et al. Restless legs syndrome symptoms in primary care: a prevalence study. Arch Intern Med 2003; 163:2323–9.
5. Phillips B, Young T, Finn L, Asher K, Hening WA, Purvis C. Epidemiology of restless legs symptoms in adults. Arch Intern Med 2000; 160:2137–41.
6. Allen RP, Picchietti D, Hening WA, Trenkwalder C, Walters AS, Montplaisir J; Restless Legs Syndrome Diagnosis and Epidemiology Workshop at the National Institutes of Health; International Restless Legs Syndrome Study Group. Restless legs syndrome: diagnostic criteria, special considerations, and epidemiology. A report from the Restless Legs Syndrome Diagnosis and Epidemiology Workshop at the National Institutes of Health. Sleep Med 2003; 4:101–19.
7. Montplaisir J, Boucher S, Poirier G, Lavigne G, Lapierre O, Lesperance P. Clinical, polysomnographic, and genetic characteristics of restless legs syndrome: a study of 133 patients diagnosed with new standard criteria. Mov Disord 1997; 12:61–5.
8. Ancoli-Israel S, Kripke DF, Klauber MR, Mason WJ, Fell R, Kaplan O. Periodic limb movements in sleep in community-dwelling elderly. Sleep 1991; 14:496–500.
9. Desautels A, Turecki G, Montplaisir J, Sequeira A, Verner A, Rouleau GA. Identification of a major susceptibility locus for restless legs syndrome on chromosome 12q. Am J Hum Genet 2001; 69:1266–70. Epub 2001 Nov 6.
10. Bonati MT, Ferini-Strambi L, Aridon P, Oldani A, Zucconi M, Casari G. Autosomal dominant restless legs syndrome maps on chromosome 14q. Brain 2003; 126(Pt 6):1485–92.
11. Chen S, Ondo WG, Rao S, Li L, Chen Q, Wang Q. Genomewide linkage scan identifies a novel susceptibility locus for restless legs syndrome on chromosome 9p. Am J Hum Genet 2004; 74:876–85. Epub 2004 Apr 7.
12. Levchenko A, Provost S, Montplaisir JY, et al. A novel autosomal dominant restless legs syndrome locus maps to chromosome 20p13. Neurology 2006; 67:900–1.
13. Pichler I, Marroni F, Volpato CB, et al. Linkage analysis identifies a novel locus for restless legs syndrome on chromosome 2q in a South Tyrolean population isolate. Am J Hum Genet 2006; 79:716–23.
14. Kemlink D, Plazzi G, Vetrugno R, et al. Suggestive evidence for linkage for restless legs syndrome on chromosome 19p13. Neurogenetics 2008; 9:75–82.
15. Winkelmann J, Schormair B, Lichtner P, et al. Genome-wide association study of restless legs syndrome identifies common variants in three genomic regions. Nat Genet 2007; 39:1000–6.
16. Stefansson H, Rye DB, Hicks A, et al. A genetic risk factor for periodic limb movements in sleep. N Engl J Med 2007; 357:639–47.
17. Schormair B, Kemlink D, Roeske D, et al. PTPRD (protein tyrosine phosphatase receptor type delta) is associated with restless legs syndrome. Nat Genet 2008; 40:946–8.
18. Sun ER, Chen CA, Ho G, Earley CJ, Allen RP. Iron and the restless legs syndrome. Sleep 1998; 21:371–7.
19. Earley CJ, Connor JR, Beard JL, Malecki EA, Epstein DK, Allen RP. Abnormalities in CSF concentrations of ferritin and transferrin in restless legs syndrome. Neurology 2000; 54:1698–700.
20. Connor JR, Boyer PJ, Menzies SL, et al. Neuropathological examination suggests impaired brain iron acquisition in restless legs syndrome. Neurology 2003; 61:304–9.
21. Silber MH, Ehrenberg BL, Allen RP, et al; Medical Advisory Board of the Restless Legs Syndrome Foundation. An algorithm for the management of restless legs syndrome. Mayo Clin Proc 2004; 79:916–22. Erratum in: Mayo Clin Proc 2004; 79: 1341.
22. Earley CJ, Horska A, Mohamed MA, Barker PB, Beard JL, Allen RP. A randomized, double-blind, placebo-controlled trial of intravenous iron sucrose in restless legs syndrome. Sleep Med. 2009; 10:206–11. Epub 2008 Feb 14.
23. Hening WA, Allen RP, Earley CJ, Picchietti DL, Silber MH; Restless Legs Syndrome Task Force of the Standards of Practice Committee of the American Academy of Sleep Medicine. An update on the dopaminergic treatment of restless legs syndrome and periodic limb movement disorder. Sleep 2004; 27:560–83.
24. García-Borreguero D, Allen RP, Benes H, et al. Augmentation as a treatment complication of restless legs syndrome: concept and management. Mov Disord 2007; 22(Suppl 18):S476–84. Erratum in: Mov Disord 2008; 23: 1200–2.
25. Tippmann-Peikert M, Park JG, Boeve BF, Shepard JW, Silber MH. Pathologic gambling in patients with restless legs syndrome treated with dopaminergic agonists. Neurology 2007; 68:301–3.
26. Man-Son-Hing M, Wells G, Lau A. Quinine for nocturnal leg cramps: a meta-analysis including unpublished data. J Gen Intern Med 1998; 13:600–6.
27. Lavigne GJ, Montplaisir JY. Restless legs syndrome and sleep bruxism: prevalence and association among Canadians. Sleep 1994; 17:739–43.
28. Ohayon MM, Li KK, Guilleminault C. Risk factors for sleep bruxism in the general population. Chest 2001; 119:53–61.
29. Aldrich MS, Jahnke B. Diagnostic value of video-EEG polysomnography. Neurology 1991; 41:1060–6.
30. Broughton RJ. Sleep disorders: disorders of arousal? Enuresis, somnambulism, and nightmares occur in confusional states of arousal, not in "dreaming sleep". Science 1968; 159:1070–8.
31. Hublin C, Kaprio J, Partinen M, Heikkila K, Koskenvuo M. Prevalence and genetics of sleepwalking: a population-based twin study. Neurology 1997; 48:177–81.
32. Ohayon MM, Guilleminault C, Priest RG. Night terrors, sleepwalking, and confusional arousals in the general population: their frequency and relationship to other sleep and mental disorders. J Clin Psychiatry 1999; 60:268–76.
33. Mahowald MW, Schenck CH, Cramer Bornemann MA. Sleep-related violence. Curr Neurol Neurosci Rep 2005; 5:153–8.
34. Bonkalo A. Impulsive acts and confusional states during incomplete arousal from sleep: crinimological and forensic implications. Psychiatr Q 1974; 48:400–9.
35. Hauri PJ, Silber MH, Boeve BF. The treatment of parasomnias with hypnosis: a 5-year follow-up study. J Clin Sleep Med 2007; 3:369–73.

36. Schenck CH, Mahowald MW. Long-term, nightly benzodiazepine treatment of injurious parasomnias and other disorders of disrupted nocturnal sleep in 170 adults. Am J Med 1996; 100:333–7.

37. Morgenthaler TI, Silber MH. Amnestic sleep-related eating disorder associated with zolpidem. Sleep Med 2002; 3:323–7.

38. Olson EJ, Boeve BF, Silber MH. Rapid eye movement sleep behaviour disorder: demographic, clinical and laboratory findings in 93 cases. Brain 2000; 123(Pt 2):331–9.

39. Schenck CH, Mahowald MW. REM sleep parasomnias. Neurol Clin 1996; 14:697–720.

40. Fantini ML, Corona A, Clerici S, Ferini-Strambi L. Aggressive dream content without daytime aggressiveness in REM sleep behavior disorder. Neurology 2005; 65:1010–5.

41. Boeve BF, Silber MH, Saper CB, et al. Pathophysiology of REM sleep behaviour disorder and relevance to neurodegenerative disease. Brain 2007; 130(Pt 11):2770–88. Epub 2007 Apr 5.

42. Gagnon JF, Bedard MA, Fantini ML, et al. REM sleep behavior disorder and REM sleep without atonia in Parkinson's disease. Neurology 2002; 59:585–9.

43. Plazzi G, Corsini R, Provini F, et al. REM sleep behavior disorders in multiple system atrophy. Neurology 1997; 48:1094–7.

44. Tachibana N, Kimura K, Kitajima K, Shinde A, Kimura J, Shibasaki H. REM sleep motor dysfunction in multiple system atrophy: with special emphasis on sleep talk as its early clinical manifestation. J Neurol Neurosurg Psychiatry 1997; 63:678–81.

45. Schenck CH, Bundlie SR, Mahowald MW. REM behavior disorder (RBD): delayed emergences of Parkinsonism and/or dementia in 65% of older men initially diagnosed with idiopathic RBD, and an analysis of the minimum and maximum tonic and/or phasic electromyographic abnormalities found during REM sleep [abstract]. Sleep 2003; 26: A316.

46. Uchiyama M, Isse K, Tanaka K, et al. Incidental Lewy body disease in a patient with REM sleep behavior disorder. Neurology 1995; 45:709–12.

47. Albin RL, Koeppe RA, Chervin RD, et al. Decreased striatal dopaminergic innervation in REM sleep behavior disorder. Neurology 2000; 55:1410–2.

48. Tippmann-Peikert M, Boeve BF, Keegan BM. REM sleep behavior disorder initiated by acute brainstem multiple sclerosis. Neurology 2006; 66:1277–9.

49. Boeve BF, Silber MH, Ferman TJ. Melatonin for treatment of REM sleep behavior disorder in neurologic disorders: results in 14 patients. Sleep Med 2003; 4:281–4.

50. Kunz D, Bes F. Melatonin as a therapy in REM sleep behavior disorder patients: an open-labeled pilot study on the possible influence of melatonin on REM-sleep regulation. Mov Disord 1999; 14:507–11.

51. Takeuchi N, Uchimura N, Hashizume Y, et al. Melatonin therapy for REM sleep behavior disorder. Psychiatry Clin Neurosci 2001; 55:267–9.

52. Schenck CH, Hurwitz TD, O'Connor KA, Mahowald MW. Additional categories of sleep-related eating disorders and the current status of treatment. Sleep 1993; 16:457–66.

53. Vetrugno R, Manconi M, Ferini-Strambi L, Provini F, Plazzi G, Montagna P. Nocturnal eating: sleep-related eating disorder or night eating syndrome? A videopolysomnographic study. Sleep 2006; 29:949–54.

54. Winkelman JW. Treatment of nocturnal eating syndrome and sleep-related eating disorder with topiramate. Sleep Med 2003; 4:243–6.

55. Pevernagie DA, Boon PA, Mariman AN, Verhaeghen DB, Pauwels RA. Vocalization during episodes of prolonged expiration: a parasomnia related to REM sleep. Sleep Med 2001; 2:19–30.

56. Vetrugno R, Provini F, Plazzi G, Vignatelli L, Lugaresi E, Montagna P. Catathrenia (nocturnal groaning): a new type of parasomnia. Neurology 2001; 56:681–3.

57. Silber MH, Hansen MR, Girish M. Complex nocturnal visual hallucinations. Sleep Med 2005; 6:363–6.

10

Circadian Rhythm Sleep Disorders: Physiology of the Circadian Clock

Lois E. Krahn, MD

ABBREVIATIONS

ASPT, advanced sleep phase type

CRSD, circadian rhythm sleep disorder

DSPT, delayed sleep phase type

FRT, free-running type

ISWT, irregular sleep-wake type

MSLT, multiple sleep latency test

REM, rapid eye movement

SCN, suprachiasmatic nuclei

VPLO, ventrolateral preoptic nuclei

Healthy sleep requires not only a sufficient quality and quantity of sleep but also sleep that occurs at the desirable time. The timing of sleep has long been known to be controlled by the interplay of circadian, homeostatic, and environmental factors. Newer findings (1) have pointed to mutations in the genes that control the human clock and to increased recognition of cultural practices as additional influences.

In recent years considerable progress in molecular genetics has been made, particularly in understanding the physiology of the human circadian clock. Chapter 1 includes an overview of the mechanisms that control the periodic transition from wakefulness to sleep. The circadian clock, which is located in the suprachiasmatic nuclei (SCN), is part of a network of hormonal and neurochemical influences. Quiescent during the day and active at night, SCN cells communicate with the nuclei of the dorsolateral hypothalamus. In turn these neurons regulate sleep by stimulating hypocretin cells in the lateral hypothalamus, leading to wakefulness by inhibiting the ventrolateral preoptic nuclei (VPLO) cells. The SCN also determines arousal by interacting with the locus coeruleus, whose cells trigger wakefulness and prevent sleep (2). Light stimulating the photoreceptors of the retina creates a signal to the pineal gland that is transmitted through noradrenergic pathways. Through this mechanism, light of sufficient intensity, especially of the blue wavelength, interferes with the pineal gland that produces melatonin long known to influence sleep onset. However, the degree to which melatonin actually regulates circadian rhythms or simply serves as a circadian marker is unknown.

In healthy human beings, the SCN has a circadian rhythm of 24.3 hours, rather than precisely 24 hours (3). This slightly longer rhythm predisposes the sleep-wake schedule to be progressively delayed (Figure 1). The circadian rhythm modulates the propensity to fall asleep, which is also determined by the duration of wakefulness, a homeostatic factor. The duration of wakefulness is controlled by intrinsic neurochemical factors such as adenosine and histamine, as well as by exogenous influences such as specific stimulating substances (e.g., caffeine or nicotine). Compared with circadian and homeostatic factors, environmental factors have been researched less but there is agreement that they also play a key role in the timing of sleep (1).

ENVIRONMENTAL FACTORS: SCHEDULES AND TIMEKEEPING

The schedules and activities of people are not dictated simply by the human need for sufficient sleep. If sleep was the only concern, a person's existence could revolve around going to sleep and awakening on demand by keying in to light in the form of sunset and dawn as time cues. Since awakening would occur naturally, there would be no need for clocks or timekeeping because the rising sun would serve this purpose. Nonetheless, for millennia other priorities have existed that require some means of timekeeping other than solar time, including the need to procure food, maintain a safe shelter, and interact with others.

Different tools have been developed over the centuries to keep time to allow people the ability to communicate with each other and coordinate activities and schedules. Communities have put particular effort into discovering or developing tools that assist with awakening. Historically, sunlight or its absence was essential to determining the passage of time. Sunrise indicated the start of the day and sunset the end; people awoke and arose and also went to bed accordingly. Animals, particularly roosters, who are alerted by the sun, created wake-up sounds. However, over the course of a year, the duration of daylight varies markedly in the higher latitudes. In Glasgow, Scotland, for example, sunset in the winter occurs in the early evening, well before most adults might complete their goals for the day. Thus artificial light in the form of candles and oil lamps was created and used worldwide to extend the workday. Communities employed lamplighters to light and extinguish lights at specified time (Figure 2). At even higher latitudes, such as the polar regions, daylight lasts for 24 hours during the summer, which necessitated the modification of dwellings to block out sunlight during the day and night. The timing and duration of sleep in such locales must be determined by factors other than the presence or absence of sunlight.

Technological advances have also evolved to assist with tracking time and alerting people to its passage. Sundials were

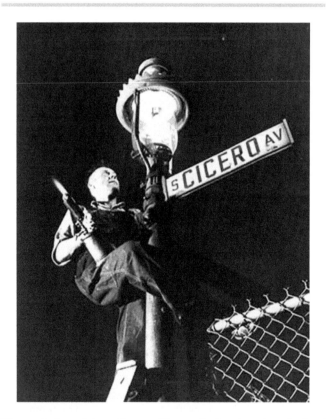

Figure 1 Delaying or Advancing Sleep. When a person needs to adapt to a new sleep schedule, it is best to gradually delay sleep (phase delay) until later rather than moving sleep forward (phase advance). (From Silber MH, Krahn LE, Morgenthaler TI. Sleep Medicine in Clinical Practice. New York: Taylor & Francis, 2004. [Used with permission of Mayo Foundation for Medical Education and Research.])

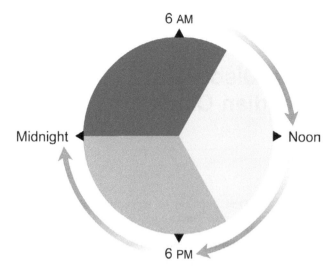

Figure 2 Lamplighter. Communities gradually adopted methods of artificial means of illumination that permitted more activities after sunset. Manually lit gasoline street lamps, such as the one shown in this 1947 photograph of a Chicago lamplighter, were used before the introduction of electricity. (From General Electric. [Used with permission.])

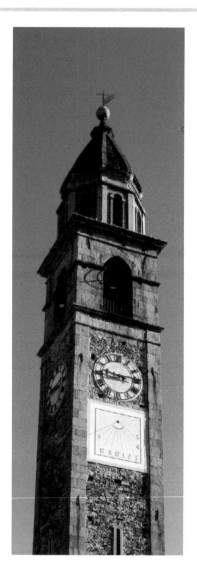

Figure 3 Clock With Its Precursor, the Sundial. Sundials such as the one on this clock tower in Ascona, Switzerland, were used to keep time before the development of reliable watches and clocks and the widespread acceptance of standard time zones. Bells sounded the time for those in the surrounding area. (Courtesy of Eric A. Gordon, Scottsdale, Arizona. [Used with permission.])

used initially, but these required a cloudless day and placement unobstructed by buildings (Figure 3). Churches, schools, and other community buildings often featured bells placed in conspicuous bell towers to help signal the time of day. One of the earliest public time systems was established in 1829 in Portsmouth, England, when a time ball was dropped from a height to signal midday. The time ball (Figure 4) instrument triggered a flag that was devised to maximize visibility from a distance so marine navigational equipment could be calibrated (4). This tradition of dropping a ball to signify the passage of time continues as a part of the annual New Year's Eve celebration in Times Square, New York City, New York. No consistent system existed to synchronize time, so church bells announcing a specific time in one community might ring minutes before or after those in a neighboring community.

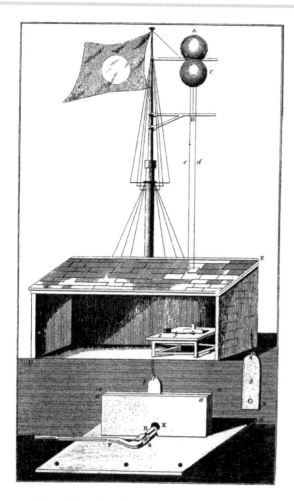

Figure 4 One of the First Time Balls. Time balls have been used since the 1800s to signal time change, with the most famous one being used on New Year's Eve in Time Squares in New York City to signal the transition to the new year. By 1833 in Greenwich, England, this technology was adopted to communicate specific times across long distances to ships. (From Bartky and Dick [4]. [Used with permission.])

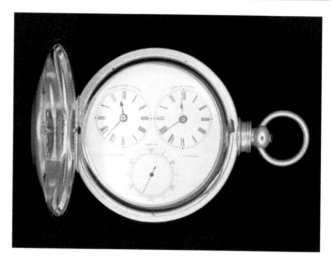

Figure 5 Double-Time Pocket Watch. The double-time watch (circa 1850) with two clock faces showing local time and railroad time side by side was used to coordinate times from region to region prior to the adoption of time zones. (From National Museum of American History, Smithsonian Institution, Washington, DC. [Used with permission.])

A coordinated system of timekeeping did not exist until 1879 when Canadian engineer Sanford Fleming proposed 24 time zones that would span the globe (5). In 1884 the International Meridian Conference in Washington, DC, was attended by 41 delegates from 25 countries who adopted this standardization, and Greenwich, England, was selected as the prime meridian, with the adjacent meridians progressively – 1 hour to the east and +1 hour to the west. Previously, every community developed its own arrangement for time, with noon being marked by the point when the sun was at its zenith overhead. Clocks were set differently in each city. This arrangement proved particularly problematic for the railroads in maintaining a consistent schedule across geographic regions. Every railway company used a company-specific measurement ("railroad time"), which was based on the time in the major hub of that company. Needless to say, railroad time was not conducive to efficient interstate commerce because it differed from local time (Figure 5). According to the *Chicago Tribune*, in the 1850s there were 27 different time zones within the state of Illinois alone (6). By 1883 the railroad companies in the eastern United

States sought a solution and agreed to "Philadelphia time," with noon in the Philadelphia region as the reference point. This led to the establishment of several time systems (Philadephia, New York, Chicago, Detroit, and Columbus time) that were not coordinated. These arrangements promoted agreement among communities within each region to synchronize their local time, but some communities, such as major metropolitan areas extending into two time zones, exerted their right to vary the boundaries in a limited way to select their own time zone. The result is a matrix of fairly irregular time zone boundaries that are influenced by both local and national considerations. As radio and television broadcasting emerged, the need for time zones became even more compelling to allow listeners to tune in to specific programs. Together with the implementation of worldwide time zones (Figure 6), rapid travel by air led to a new cause of sleep disruption. Travelers making transmeridian trips, either from west to east or vice versa, must adjust their sleep-wake schedule to accommodate to the time at their destination. Jet lag will be discussed in more depth later in the chapter.

Daylight saving time, adopted in early 1918 by the U.S. Congress with its passage of the Standard Time Act to boost manufacturing production during wartime, represents another level of complexity (Figure 7). Many jurisdictions worldwide currently agree to move clocks forward by one hour in the summer to ensure that there are more daylight hours in the morning than in the afternoon. However, even this modest advance in time has been linked in several countries with a surge in motor vehicle accidents, presumably due to decreased alertness and fatigue caused by incomplete adaptation to the new time (7).

CIRCADIAN RHYTHM SLEEP DISORDERS

In the absence of an alarm clock, persons will conceivably awaken after they have obtained sufficient sleep. Factors that contribute to the timing of sleep include total sleep time and

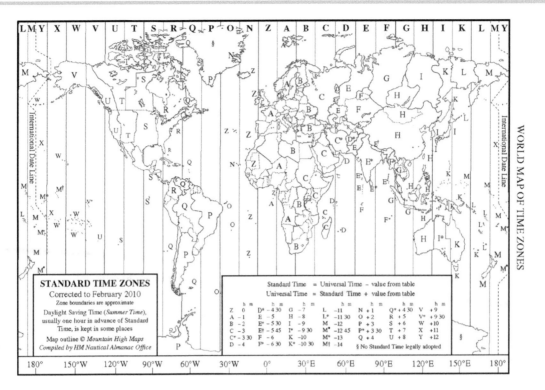

Figure 6 Standard Time Zones Around the World. A system of 24 time zones spaced at intervals of 15° longitude representing 1-hour time intervals was adopted worldwide in the late 1800s to coordinate transportation and communication. Letter key indicates times east or west of the prime meridian (universal time [Greenwich mean time]), with 1 hour plus (to east) or 1 hour minus (to west) for each time zone. (From HM Nautical Almanac Office, Taunton, England, United Kingdom. [Used with permission.])

accumulated sleep debt (homeostatic), time of sleep onset, core body temperature, conditioned awakening (circadian), genetic mutations (8), and exposure to sunlight, noise, and vibration (environmental). Other significant contributors include cultural factors, such as the practice of the siesta. The circadian rhythm sleep disorders (CRSD) are defined as a persistent pattern of sleep disturbances primarily caused by alterations in circadian timekeeping that lead to impairment (Table 1; Figure 8). In clinical populations the most common type of CRSD is delayed sleep phase type (DSPT), which represented 83% of the identified cases in one study (9).

Free-Running Type

Free-running type (FRT) sleep disorder, a type of CRSD also known as non–24-hour sleep-wake disorder or hypernychthemeral disorder, is diagnosed in patients lacking an entrained sleep rhythm. The medical and social consequences of FRT have not been well studied but might be expected to include family and professional difficulties.

This condition, which is rare in persons with normal vision, is most often detected in blind patients, 50% of whom have it (10). These patients cannot benefit from the powerful entraining effect of light on the SCN and instead experience a free-running rhythm without a consistent sleep phase. Clinically, such patients may present with intermittent insomnia and excessive daytime sleepiness. Although their sleep-wake activity may briefly be synchronized with that of the community where they reside, it will again drift out of phase after

several days. The observed sleep patterns of persons with FRT CRSD are similar to those seen in subjects living without environmental time cues. Other unpredictable circadian rhythms may also develop, and melatonin secretion will no longer be synchronized with the sleep-wake pattern when it is irregular. Patients complain of undesired daytime sleepiness corresponding to diurnal melatonin that is not suppressed in the absence of light perception (11). In a process of internal desynchronization, the sleep-wake rhythm dissociates from the body's other circadian rhythms, such as temperature, cortisol, and melatonin. Difficulty in initiating sleep may be exacerbated when the FRT for sleep-wake activity corresponds to points on the temperature rhythm other than the nadir.

When FRT is identified in persons with normal retinal function, psychiatric difficulties are also often present (12). In such circumstances, FRT must be distinguished from irregular sleep-wake type (ISWT). Actigraphy and sleep logs can be helpful in documenting a non–24-hour sleep rhythm. Treatment depends on whether patients have functioning retinas. Melatonin levels and core body temperatures can be used as markers of circadian phase. Social or cultural cues are especially important because phototherapy is generally unsuccessful in patients with neurological impairment. Timed administration of melatonin is useful for moving blind patients along in a carefully planned sleep-wake schedule. For those rare patients with intact vision who have non–24-hour sleep rhythm, light exposure may be a useful addition to melatonin and to a prescribed sleep schedule.

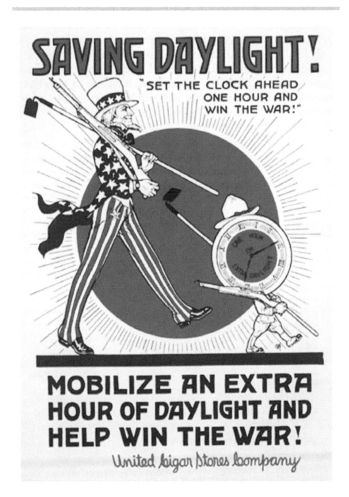

Figure 7 Poster Promoting Daylight Saving Time. "Saving Daylight" poster (circa 1918) publicized the idea of advancing the clock in the spring for the summer months nationwide in the United States during World War I to boost productivity as part of the war effort. (From Warshaw Collection of Business Americana, National Museum of American History, Smithsonian Institution, Washington, DC. [Used with permission.])

Table 1 Classification of the circadian rhythm sleep disorders

Disorders with persistent misalignment to time due to intrinsic
    factors related to time in the community
        Free-running type (FRT)
        Irregular sleep-wake type (ISWT)
        Delayed sleep phase type (DSPT)
        Advanced sleep phase type (ASPT)
Disorders resulting from imposed or voluntary shifts in the timing of
    sleep due to external factors that lead to an incomplete adaptation
        Jet lag type
        Shift work type

Data from The International Classification of Sleep Disorders: Diagnostic and Coding Manual. 2nd ed. Westchester (IL): American Academy of Sleep Medicine, 2005. Used with permission.

One recent sleep study used polysomnography, actigraphy, and Braille sleep logs to examine the sleep of 26 totally blind patients and 26 matched controls (13). These patients were living in the community but had multiple sleep complaints,

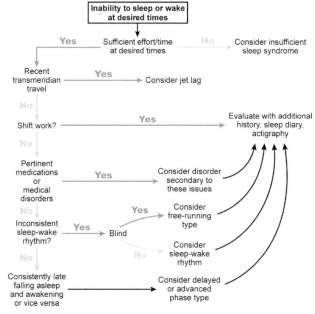

Diagnostic Algorithm for Circadian Rhythm Sleep Disorders

Figure 8 Diagnostic Algorithm for Circadian Sleep Disorders. This flow chart indicates the sequential order of the issues that should be considered when a clinician assesses a patient with a potential circadian rhythm sleep disorder.

presumably due to an FRT cycle. Patients who were employed had a longer major sleep period than those who were retired or unemployed. Similarly, in my experience, patients with FRT who are mentally retarded may cope more poorly because of increased difficulty in conforming to social routines.

Free-running type should be suspected in any patient without light perception who has sleep complaints. The medical and social consequences of FRT have not been well studied but might be expected to include family and professional difficulties. FRT should be differentiated from the other circadian rhythm disorders, including DSPT. Patients with DSPT initially have insomnia. In contrast to non–24-hour sleep-wake rhythm disorder, DSPT patients experience a stable sleep-wake cycle, albeit delayed, sometimes to an extreme degree. Irregular sleep-wake type is another diagnostic consideration. Patients with an inconsistent sleep-wake schedule are capable of entrainment but disregard the cues. A detailed sleep diary recording several weeks of functioning, accompanied by wrist actigraphy, can assist in distinguishing among these syndromes.

Few studies have examined therapeutic options. Melatonin has been explored as a means to entrain circadian rhythms. Low-dose (0.5 mg) melatonin is typically administered at 8 PM (expected to be near the time of melatonin onset), provided a person is in dim light to achieve an effect by 11 PM (14). A sleep diary should be used initially, with melatonin treatment beginning only after the major sleep period occurs at night. Despite the absence of sight in blind persons, it is worthwhile to assess whether bright light suppresses melatonin because the retino-hypothalamic pathway occasionally remains intact. In such cases, bright light may be used for entrainment. Since FRT is typically a lifelong disorder, other environmental cues such as social activities and exercise also have enhanced therapeutic value.

Irregular Sleep-Wake Type

Patients with ISWT have the capacity for entrainment yet fail to develop a consistent sleep-wake rhythm. They lack the normal sleep-wake pattern of a major sleep period, possibly with a secondary nap in the early afternoon. Instead, their sleep is randomly scattered and interspersed with wakefulness throughout the 24-hour day (Figure 9). This disorder evolves

from poor sleep hygiene. Patients may be unable to adhere to a more consistent sleep-wake cycle because of dementia or mental retardation (15). Whether SCN function is normal in patients with ISWT is unknown because little research has been conducted on patients with this type of sleep disorder. Patients at higher risk of ISWT are older and have more psychiatric problems (16). Many elderly patients have dementia and live in institutional settings where they are less likely to be exposed to sunlight during the day. Alzheimer disease and related disorders may be associated with degenerative retinal changes. Actigraphy and/or a sleep diary can be extremely helpful in documenting this irregular sleep pattern.

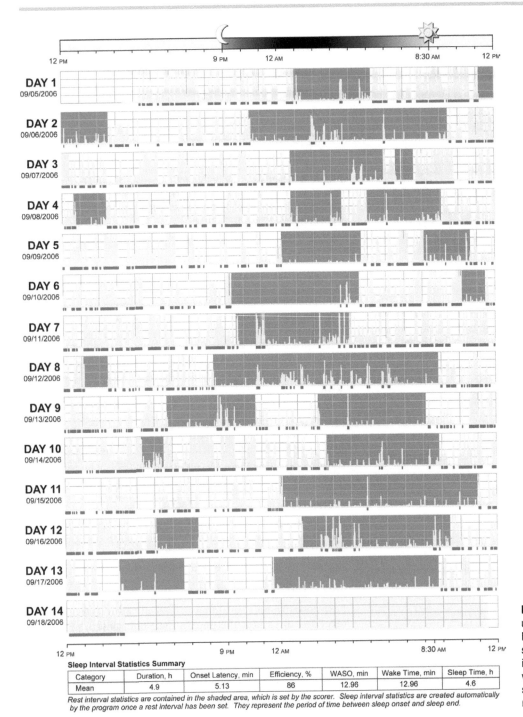

Figure 9 Wrist Actigraphy of Irregular Sleep-Wake Type Circadian Rhythm Disorder. This patient had substantial social isolation and coexisting obsessive-compulsive disorder, which contributed to the irregular sleep-wake pattern. WASO, wakefulness after sleep onset.

Sleep Interval Statistics Summary

Category	Duration, h	Onset Latency, min	Efficiency, %	WASO, min	Wake Time, min	Sleep Time, h
Mean	4.9	5.13	86	12.96	12.96	4.6

Rest interval statistics are contained in the shaded area, which is set by the scorer. Sleep interval statistics are created automatically by the program once a rest interval has been set. They represent the period of time between sleep onset and sleep end.

Treatment for ISWT involves striving to establish a more conventional circadian rhythm of sleep-wake activity. This can be pursued by enhancing cues to sleep and awaken. Research results have been inconsistent, but exposure to bright morning light has been found to improve the quantity of nighttime sleep if not wakefulness. Melatonin has been tried but the results of such studies have been conflicting. Hypnotic agents should be used with caution because of the risk of aggravating preexisting cognitive impairment. Patient education in sleep hygiene and daily physical activity to establish a daily routine are safe and likely beneficial.

Delayed Sleep Phase Type

Patients with DSPT fall asleep later and awaken later than expected or desired. This disorder may be quite common, although in-depth epidemiological studies are lacking. In one study of 10,000 Scandinavians followed with sleep logs, a prevalence of 0.72% was reported (17). This number is probably an underestimate because of the limitations of survey research and because few affected people will actually seek treatment for DSPT. The mean age of onset is 15 years. Although DSPT is a chronic condition, it rarely starts after 30 years of age so is seldom seen in older persons. Some studies report a male predominance, but the mix by sex is uncertain (18). There are fewer reports of a familial predisposition for DSPT than there are for advanced sleep phase type (ASPT) sleep disorder. Genetic studies of familial DSPT have revealed some intriguing clues; for example, there may be an autosomal dominant means of inheritance with incomplete penetrance (19). A higher than expected frequency of hPer3, an abnormality of the period (*Per3*) gene that influences the circadian period, has been observed (20,21). Studies of patients with a propensity for eveningness (the natural propensity to be active in the evening vs in the morning) but lacking a familial predisposition have revealed alterations in the *CLOCK* gene but have identified no specific polymorphism (22,23).

DSPT is relatively common in adolescents, possibly because persons in this developmental stage of maturation have the highest propensity to delay going to sleep by staying up late and then to extend the time to awakening by sleeping in. Mechanisms that explain the higher rate of DSPT during adolescence include a longer circadian period or reduced sensitivity to light. These two factors may be intertwined because adolescents who sleep late into the morning have less opportunity for exposure to morning light with its recognized benefits in advancing sleep phase.

DSPT can have major consequences. For adolescents, arising late interferes greatly with school attendance and academic success. Over time patients may develop poor self-esteem because they are struggling not only with the academic but also with the social components of school. The high association of DSPT and depression is likely explained by the combination of sleep difficulties and the resulting frustrating school experience. Thus treatment should involve both phototherapy and psychotherapy to target both sleep and psychosocial issues.

The diagnosis of DSPT requires careful assessment of the patient's sleep-wake schedule over the course of at least one week. A sleep diary is valuable but highly dependent on patient compliance in completing the daily forms accurately and on time. Wrist actigraphy is a useful technology that detects a person's movement and, by extrapolation, the sleep-wake cycle in the home environment. Its comparison with the sleep diary permits the clinician to determine whether the patient is reliably reporting his or her sleep schedule. The self-assessment Morningness-Eveningness Questionnaire is used widely to assist in characterizing the natural propensity to be a night owl or a morning lark (24).

DSPT is characterized by initial sleep and wake times that are consistently later than desired. The total sleep time over a 24-hour period is normal. Many patients report that the problem arises after a stretch of late-night studying or social activities. Those who manage to arise at a socially acceptable hour usually experience excessive daytime sleepiness during the morning. On vacation, when they are not trying to conform to a specified schedule, their wake time will be delayed. Patients with DSPT often recognize that they have the long-standing trait of being night owls because they feel most alert and perform best late at night. Some individuals cope by selecting careers that involve evenings and avoid mornings, such as restaurant work. Students may compensate by going to night school.

DSPT is often associated with psychiatric disorders, specifically depression (25). It is unclear whether affected adolescents first have psychiatric symptoms and then develop DSPT or whether the circadian rhythm disorder leads to absenteeism which, in turn, results in psychiatric, academic, and social problems. Patients and their families are often intensely frustrated by the condition.

The differential diagnosis includes major depression in patients with DSPT who have an increased need to sleep that sometimes coexists with an initial insomnia. If a patient pursues treatment for the mood disorder and has improvement in mood and other symptoms but persistent delayed sleep phase, then a coexisting CRSD should be suspected. Some patients with avoidant or schizoid personality disorder will seek out the solitude of night. A careful history taking not only should explore the person's sleep-wake schedule but also should look for signs of deliberate avoidance of daytime interactions. Some people who are disabled, unemployed, or on vacation may voluntarily select a late-night schedule. Determining the motivation and effort expended to conform to the more conventional timetable can help differentiate them from true DSPT patients.

Patients with DSPT will occasionally appear to have a disorder of excessive daytime sleepiness such as narcolepsy or idiopathic hypersomnia. Thus assessment should include careful exploration for the presence of excessive sleepiness during the evening and night because normal alertness during these times more likely indicates DSPT. Patients with DSPT may have periods of sleep-onset rapid eye movement (REM) during the first or second naps of the multiple sleep latency test (MSLT), especially if the MSLT start time was not delayed in accordance with the patient's phase shift. The finding of REM sleep in an early MSLT nap would not reflect REM sleep intruding into daytime alertness but rather the patient's final REM sleep of the major sleep period. Initial sleep latency usually increases with successive naps in DSPT. For all the CRSD, polysomnography may be indicated if there is any suspicion of a coexisting sleep disorder such as obstructive sleep apnea. When polysomnography is used, the start time of the sleep study may have to be adjusted.

Patients must strive toward a consistent sleep-wake schedule because deliberately staying up late on weekends and holidays can interfere with falling asleep as desired on weeknights (26). Patient motivation is an essential component in a successful treatment plan. If the patient does not actively embrace the practices necessary to correct the CRSD, then treatment is unlikely to be effective. In some cases a patient may espouse an intention to strive for a phase shift but actually maintain a passive-aggressive attitude that can contribute significantly to family strain. Thus in many cases psychotherapy may be essential to give the patient an opportunity to understand and modify the factors that may be contributing to sleep-interfering activities engaged in late at night. Family therapy as well as individual therapy may be useful in finding solutions to complex family and school problems.

The most commonly recommended treatment for DSPT is to have patients use bright-light therapy in the morning from 6 AM to 9 AM to adjust the sleep-wake cycle. When patients adhere to this approach, it can be effective. Patients typically start at a later time (e.g., 9 AM) and advance the time of light exposure as their ability to awake earlier improves. However, adherence to these procedures is difficult because patients are typically more pressed for time in the morning, and many patients have difficulty awakening earlier just for the purpose of getting light exposure from a light box or the sun. Adherence is often inconsistent, with patients complaining that they cannot find the necessary 30 minutes each morning for the treatment.

The light intensity used in clinical trials has been 2,500 to 25,000 lux (26,27). Several different light units are available and the manufacturers' specifications should be followed concerning the distance for the patient to sit from the light box. The distance varies, depending on whether the unit has a single central light or two smaller units that are placed on either side of the patient. Patients should make light exposure their priority and should engage in activities such as reading, applying makeup, or eating breakfast only if their eyes are positioned adequately in front of the box. Many patients prefer to combine their exposure to natural sunshine with exercise by jogging, biking, or running outside in clear weather. To prevent eye damage, patients should never look directly at the sun. Potential side effects of light boxes include retinal burns, which are more likely to develop if the patient is taking anticholinergic medications that increase pupillary diameter (28). Patients taking photosensitizing medications should not be advised to use phototherapy.

Patients with DSPT should also be advised to avoid bright light, possibly by wearing sunglasses, from 4 PM to dark. Other treatment options have included the use of melatonin, which has been beneficial in several controlled trials (29–31). Melatonin should be taken one to three hours (depending on the severity of the phase delay) before the desired bedtime and it should continue to be used on an ongoing basis. The dose of melatonin is typically low (3 mg). Melatonin has not been tested as rigorously for side effects as have hypnotic agents. Since it is not considered a pharmaceutical agent by the U.S. Food and Drug Administration but rather is classified as a nutritional supplement available in health food stores, patients may have difficulty verifying the purity of the product available for purchase. Safety data regarding the long-term use of melatonin have not appeared in the medical literature, although no anecdotal reports of serious side effects have surfaced to date. In general, melatonin is only weakly sedating. Some experts advocate combining melatonin with phototherapy (32). This combined approach may be desirable when patients are suspected of having poor adherence with phototherapy and would be more likely to take a tablet. Apart from the increased cost, there are no known risks to combining melatonin with light therapy.

Most treatment plans for DSPT no longer emphasize the role of chronotherapy. Using this approach, patients in one study sequentially delayed their bedtime by one to two hours a night around the clock until they finally could fall asleep at the desired time (33). Outcomes were poor because of the understandable difficulty in conforming to this complex regimen and the tendency for many patients to slip back into a DSPT pattern over time. Hypnosis and psychostimulants have not been found to be useful because patients fundamentally get adequate sleep but are not synchronized with their community. If the patient has coexisting major depression, antidepressant medication may be appropriate. Some clinicians opt to prescribe sedating antidepressants such as mirtazapine, although these medications have not been demonstrated to be preferable to agents that are not sedating.

Advanced Sleep Phase Type

Patients with ASPT fall asleep and awaken at earlier times than desired and may inappropriately fall asleep during evening activities. While awake in the early morning, they may experience loneliness or boredom. The condition is thought to be rare, although its incidence may be underestimated since patients may not recognize or report this problem to their physician. The institutional routines in nursing homes and assisted living facilities frequently encourage bedtime in the early evening, sometimes because of reduced staffing at those times.

A survey of 10,000 Scandinavians did not identify a single case of ASPT (17). This condition is thought to be markedly less common than DSPT because the period of the human circadian rhythm is slightly longer than 24 hours, which makes it easier to stay up late than to fall asleep earlier. The condition likely becomes more common with age. ASPT may be more common in older adults because they often live in institutional settings that reinforce an earlier bedtime. The striking difference in prevalence between ASPT and DSPT is likely because the human sleep-wake circadian period of slightly more than 24 hours promotes phase delay.

The diagnostic evaluation for ASPT is the same as that for DSPT. Unless the clinician is aware of the timing of the patient's major sleep period, this condition may be mistaken for a disorder of excessive daytime sleepiness because those affected with ASPT can fall asleep during evening activities or can experience insomnia due to prior wakefulness during the latter part of the night. Major depression is another important part of the differential diagnosis because early morning insomnia can be observed in both conditions.

ASPT has provided an invaluable clue to the genetics of the mechanisms controlling sleep-wake behavior. Patients in four families were studied and all of those affected fell asleep four hours earlier and also awakened earlier than expected (8). The melatonin levels and temperature rhythms of these patients were advanced by three to four hours. Their circadian sleep-wake period was shortened to 23.3 hours. An autosomal dominant familial form of ASPT was identified. The genetic defect was traced to hPer2, a mutation in the Per2 gene. Affected individuals have a mutation in the casein kinase 1–binding region of the hPer2 gene with a serine to glycine mutation. This mutation interferes with the functioning of the CLOCK component, which causes a significant advance in the circadian period that is consistent with ASPT (8).

Most research on the treatment of ASPT has focused on the role of light in shifting the sleep-wake rhythm. Treatment involves avoidance of morning bright light and implementation of a daytime schedule that encourages entrainment to a conventional sleep-wake schedule. Evening light therapy has also been successfully used in short-term studies (34,35). Progressive earlier shifting of bedtime by three hours every two days has been reported as having short-term utility in several cases (34,35). One recent study examined therapy of ASPT in a group of children with Smith-Magenis syndrome, a complex genetic disease caused by a deletion in chromosome 17p (36). Sleep, as well as melatonin phase, was delayed with the administration in the evening of controlled-release melatonin combined with administration in the morning of a β_1-adrenergic antagonist to block the noradrenergic neurotransmission to the pineal gland that releases melatonin (34,35).

Jet Lag Type

With the development of long-distance transmeridian travel, a new sleep disorder has emerged. Jet lag type (otherwise known as time zone change syndrome) represents an acute problem in which the sleep-wake circadian rhythms of travelers become out of phase with the light-dark cycle at their destination. The magnitude of the problem increases as travelers cross more time zones. In general, without measures to accelerate adjustment, one day must lapse to adjust to every hour of time zone change. Longitudinal (north-south) air travel may result in sleep debt related to the inability to obtain quality sleep while aboard an airplane, but it does not challenge travelers in the same fashion by requiring them to adapt to a new time zone.

The entrainment process is facilitated for travelers with jet lag as they attempt to adapt to the sleep-wake cycle of the destination community. Most people can more readily phase delay than they can phase advance the timing of their major sleep period, probably because of the longer than 24-hour periodicity of the human circadian pacemaker. Thus east to west travel is typically easier to adjust to than the equivalent travel west to east. Travelers who make frequent long-distance trips can develop a chronic condition of jet lag when they do not adequately adapt before a further change in sleep-wake schedule is required. For travelers such as airline personnel who face frequent circadian adjustments because of their work schedules, jet lag overlaps with shift work sleep disorder.

The consequences of jet lag are similar to those of other CRSDs: excessive daytime sleepiness, insomnia, disturbed nocturnal sleep, and occupational problems due to inadequate alertness (Figure 10). The effect of jet lag on other circadian rhythms is less well known. Some travelers tolerate transmeridian travel without significant jet lag, but the reasons for individual variations are not well understood. There are no known differences in jet lag by sex, but there is a decrease with age in the ability to adjust sleep-wake rhythms. Treatment options are controversial and no one strategy is clearly preferred. Numerous research studies have been conducted on jet lag but most have significant limitations, primarily due to study design issues such as the inability to control light exposure or to ensure subject adherence with the protocol. Few experimental models exist for jet lag that account for all the variables encountered in the real world of travel. For example, one protocol might call for three successive days of exposure to bright light at a consistent time for approximately 3 hours after arrival at a destination, which might not be feasible for most tourists or business travelers.

The most commonly used strategies are optimization of sleep hygiene, manipulation of the sleep-wake schedule, use of melatonin, use of phototherapy, and the judicious use of caffeinated beverages and foods or hypnotics. A daytime flight eliminates the need for adequate sleep in an uncomfortable setting. Helpful measures at the destination include using a bedroom that is dark and quiet, and of a comfortable temperature. Relaxation techniques such as diaphragmatic breathing or progressive muscle relaxation may hasten sleep onset at an unfamiliar hour. The use of alcohol is not recommended. Dietary measures have been proposed, such as a presleep tryptophan-rich carbohydrate diet (promoting sedation mediated by serotonin and therefore initiating melatonin production) and protein intake upon awakening (increasing alertness by means of tyrosine), but these programs are not supported by convincing evidence. Herbal remedies, other than melatonin, are of limited usefulness.

One practical approach is to try to adapt the time of the major sleep period as quickly as possible to the new schedule. For example, if a traveler arrives at 6 AM in Europe after a west to east trans-Atlantic flight, that person is phase delayed by as much as six or seven hours behind the time at the destination. For example, the traveler's sleep-wake rhythm may be at 1 to 2 AM when the morning activities start in Europe. The traveler could stay awake all day, causing an abrupt advance in sleep phase by avoiding sleep until as close as possible to the desired bedtime. For westward flights, the circadian challenge is the opposite. Such persons need to adapt to their advanced sleep phase by phase delaying their sleep-wake schedule to conform to the time at their destination.

Meals and exercise at the destination should be timed carefully to serve as social cues that encourage and reinforce an appropriate sleep-wake cycle. Some experts advocate naps before, during, and after transmeridian travel to prevent development of a substantial sleep debt. These naps should be timed carefully to allow sufficient sleep pressure to build up so that the traveler can still initiate sleep at the desired bedtime at the destination. Caffeine use should be carefully tracked so as to minimize caffeine-related insomnia. In moderation, caffeine can be used to enhance alertness. Armodafinil, an isomer of modafinil approved for treatment of excessive sleepiness due to obstructive sleep apnea, shift work disorder, or narcolepsy, has been studied for jet lag disorder (37) but was not approved by the U.S. Food and Drug Administration for that indication in a March 2010 decision.

Hypnotics, traditionally the short-acting benzodiazepines such as triazolam, have been shown to be of some benefit in treating jet lag. These compounds decrease sleep latency, reduce awakenings, and increase total sleep time. Nonbenzodiazepine agents with short half-lives (e.g., zolpidem, zaleplon, and zopiclone) are a more recently available but less studied option. The half-life of any hypnotic should be short to avoid a hangover effect. Potential side effects of both classes of hypnotics include amnesia, and cognitive impairment may occur with benzodiazepines.

Since bright light is known to exert the strongest influence on the SCN, this modality has clear potential for resetting the sleep-wake circadian rhythm to match the schedule at the destination. Numerous studies have led to jet lag algorithms. If a phase advance is desired, the intent is to get light exposure before the concurrent melatonin peak and temperature nadir. If a phase delay is sought, the light exposure should come after these circadian markers. Use of carefully timed light exposure

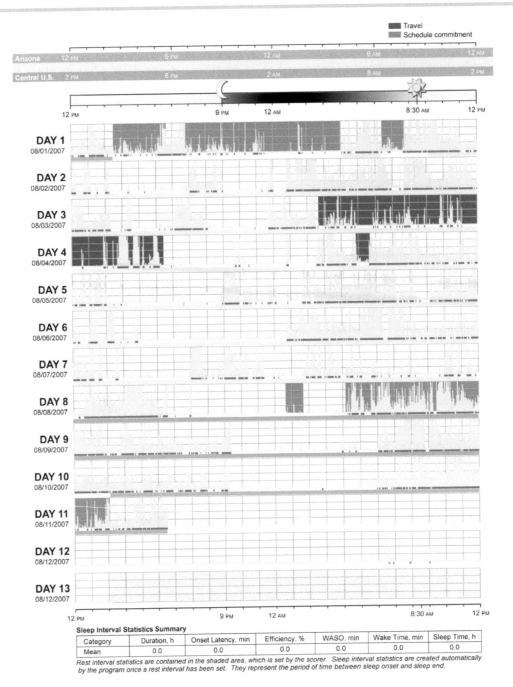

Figure 10 Wrist Actigraphy of Jet Lag. Jet lag is especially common in travelers flying between North America and Europe. WASO, wakefulness after sleep onset.

may accelerate phase adjustments from a change of one hour to a change of three hours per day. This strategy, while scientifically based on the physiology of the SCN, is difficult to implement in real-life travel. There are no simple tools for determining peak melatonin or for measuring core body temperature. In addition, the optimal duration of a session of phototherapy, the number of successive daily sessions, the light spectrum, and the effects of age and individual differences are all unknown. Nonetheless, awareness of the effects of light on circadian rhythms is important because travelers should at least avoid exposure to

bright light at critical times. If phase advance is desired, morning bright light exposure should be minimized (potentially by using wraparound sunglasses); for a desired phase delay, bright light should be avoided in the evening.

Melatonin has been the subject of intense interest as a tool for the prevention or treatment of jet lag. Some, but not all, studies show the value of this compound as a chronotherapeutic agent for subjectively improving jet lag (38,39). Melatonin should be administered at a 12-hour phase difference from light therapy. If provided before the nadir of the core body temperature, melatonin will advance the sleep-wake circadian rhythm. If administered after this pivotal point, rhythms will delay. Experts advise travelers to start using melatonin during the early evening before departure for eastward trips and thereafter at the desired bedtime at the destination. For westward travel after arrival at the destination, melatonin should be administered at 11 PM or even later to promote a phase delay.

Shift Work Type

Many occupations involve work shifts that may encompass night work, evening shifts, split 24-hour schedules, early morning start times, and on-call responsibilities (Table 2). Workers with rotating schedules are at higher risk for complications because their sleep-wake circadian rhythm is constantly adapting to a new timetable as opposed to straight second (evening) or third (night) shift (Figure 11). Workers with family or school responsibilities face even more difficulties finding adequate time to sleep (Figure 12). In general, older persons find it harder to adapt to shift changes than do younger ones.

Shift workers have high rates of both insomnia and excessive daytime sleepiness. Because of environmental factors, such as neighborhood noise or sunlight, it may be difficult to initiate or maintain sleep during the day. Many night-shift workers are chronically sleep deprived, getting as little as two to four hours of sleep, because they have difficulty sleeping during the day or end up sacrificing sleep to spend time with family, in leisure activities, or in running errands. Those with a coexisting sleep disorder, such as obstructive sleep apnea, have an increased probability of excessive daytime sleepiness. Shift

work puts persons at high risk for several problems. Working when not fully alert poses the risk of performance difficulties because of diminished vigilance. Research into fatigue reveals that patients can experience cognitive or motor impairment (40). Many devastating industrial or transportation incidents, including the Exxon Valdez oil tanker spill in Alaska in 1989 and the Three Mile Island nuclear power plant accident in Pennsylvania in 1979, have occurred at night, which suggests that worker fatigue may have been a contributing factor.

Social and medical problems are also associated with shift work. Missing opportunities to interact with family or friends because of the timing of the shift or the subsequent recovery sleep can lead to social problems and family strain. Young children in particular may have difficulty understanding that a parent must be allowed to get adequate sleep after returning home from work. One recent study found an increase in common respiratory infections and gastroenteritis in shift workers, with more in the third shift than in the second, possibly because fatigue renders employees more vulnerable to infections (41).

Several strategies have been identified to assist workers who must incorporate shift work into their lifestyle. Some people can use their affinity for functioning well at certain times; for example, people with a tendency toward a delayed sleep phase may actually cope satisfactorily with an evening work schedule, providing they can sleep in late the following morning. Meals should be timed to promote sleep. Hunger or foods that cause dyspepsia may fragment sleep. The workplace environment should be carefully planned to take into account the safety and sleep needs of workers. Bright lights and a

Table 2 Occupations frequently requiring shift work

Time of shift	Type of work or worker
Early shift	Agriculture (dairy)
	Bakeries
	Health care (surgical staff, anesthesiology)
Late shift	Restaurant (food preparation and serving)
	Entertainment (musicians, performers)
	Private security (guards, patrols)
	Custodial (janitors, after-hours construction/renovation)
	Astronomers/astrophysicists (telescope/observatory)
	Transporation (taxi, limousine)
Schedules designed to provide continuous coverage	Aviation (pilots, flight attendants, mechanics, reservations staff)
	Seafaring/nautical (captains, pilots, engineers, lighthouse)
	Information technology (help desk staff)
	Health care (physicians, nurses, pharmacists, technologists)
	Military (air traffic control, navy, combat)
	Public safety (police, firefighters, emergency medical personnel)
	Public security (coast guard, border control, airport security)
	Mining/natural resources (offshore oil rigs, mines)
	Manufacturing (assembly lines, factories)
	Retail (convenience marts, superstores)
Schedules dependent on time zone differences with other offices	Investment (stock exchanges, commodities exchanges)
	International finance
	News media deadlines
	Diplomacy/international affairs
	Multinational companies
Schedules with seasonal variation	Accountants (tax deadlines)
	Researchers (grant deadlines)
	Agriculture (planting, harvest)
	Fisheries (seasonal catches)
	Movie production (filming on location)

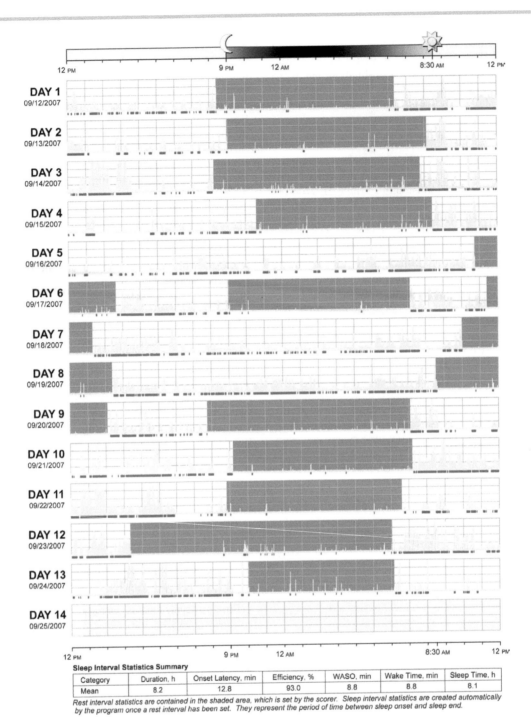

Category	Duration, h	Onset Latency, min	Efficiency, %	WASO, min	Wake Time, min	Sleep Time, h
Mean	8.2	12.8	93.0	8.8	8.8	8.1

Rest interval statistics are contained in the shaded area, which is set by the scorer. Sleep interval statistics are created automatically by the program once a rest interval has been set. They represent the period of time between sleep onset and sleep end.

Figure 11 Wrist Actigraphy of Shift Work Sleep Disorder. Registered nurses who work varying shifts (eg, nights and then days) often have shift work sleep disorder. WASO, wakefulness after sleep onset.

slightly cool air temperature may improve alertness. Ideally, attention should be given to the type of tasks undertaken by employees, especially on the night shift, with stimulating activities interspersed among monotonous duties.

Controlling light exposure is critically important. A person might wear dark glasses for the drive home from work after dawn. The sleeping environment at home might have to be modified. A quiet and dark bedroom is more important to a shift worker than to those who work day jobs. Special window coverings may be required. The telephone should be switched off and an answering machine should be used to collect messages. Family members should be reminded not to awaken the shift worker in the midst of his or her major sleep period. Sleep hygiene should be optimized in all respects.

Studies have shown that workers cope better when switching from one shift to another if they delay, rather than

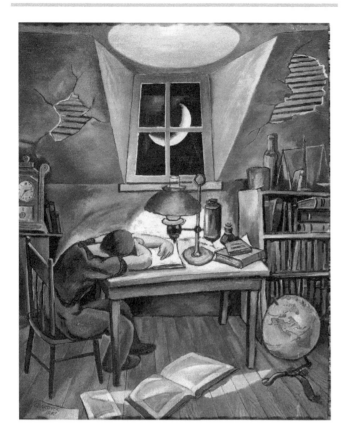

Figure 12 Delayed Sleep Phase Type of Sleep Disorder. Oil painting entitled *Poor Student* (1932) by Fred Gardner illustrates the delayed sleep phase type of sleep disorder common in adolescents. (From Smithsonian American Art Museum, Washington, DC. [Used with permission.])

as they cannot predict when they will be required to perform a task. Typically, the shifts for on-call workers are longer than those for most other shift workers (for example, the 24-hour shift common among firefighters). Sleep is encouraged and accommodations provided, but workers cannot count on being able to sleep. Under these circumstances, naps may be especially important. Although people are generally urged to have a major sleep period each 24-hour day, as opposed to several shorter stretches of sleep, naps are acceptable if they are the only means by which adequate sleep can be obtained.

Medications have been examined to help shift workers initiate sleep at the desired time (26,44). Regular use of long-acting benzodiazepines not only creates a hangover effect, especially with longer-acting agents, but also runs the risk of physical dependence. Short-term use of a newer nonbenzodiazepine hypnotic such as zaleplon or ramelteon is preferable to a benzodiazepine. Even with these agents, caution must be taken because few studies have examined their long-term use or addressed their interaction with shift work. Medications are not the first choice of intervention. First, workers should fully explore various means to get adequate sleep by making careful schedule changes, keeping sufficient sleep a priority, and taking naps as indicated. The hypnotics provide symptomatic relief without addressing the underlying circadian rhythm disturbance inherent in shift work. Alcohol should be avoided as a means of inducing sleep because of its tendency to reduce the quality of non-REM sleep and its detrimental effects on the patency of the upper airway. Caffeine may be useful to boost alertness, but it should be avoided close to bedtime because it can interfere with sleep onset. Judicious use of the alerting agent modafinil, the only medication approved by the U.S. Food and Drug Administration for managing shift work sleep disorder, is an appropriate means of treatment. Modafinil represents the compensation strategy of boosting alertness, but it carries the risk of inadequately addressing the sleep deprivation responsible for sleepiness. Bright-light therapy delivered at precise times may also be useful. Melatonin has been explored as a possible chronotherapeutic agent. More recently, the melatonin agonist ramelteon has shown promise in pilot studies but large-scale studies are not yet available (45).

advance, their work and sleep times (42). For instance, most persons who move from an evening shift to a night shift will adjust more easily to the change than if they were moving from a night shift to an evening shift. Preparing for an approaching change to a later shift by gradually moving bedtime and wake time back by two hours starting several days before the switch has been found to be beneficial. However, family responsibilities often complicate carefully planned sleep schedule adjustments of this type. Other effective coping strategies include taking a sleep break during work hours. Recent research that has focused on the transportation industry, specifically airline personnel, indicates that a 30-minute nap partway through the shift increases productivity, reduces fatigue, and improves employee satisfaction (43). Long-haul aircraft have now been designed to include bunks or reclining seats for scheduled naps.

Some employers and employees prefer work schedules that use permanent shift assignments. Night shift workers should endeavor to keep to a consistent sleep-wake schedule even on days when they do not work. Reverting to nighttime sleep over a weekend or on a single day off presents adjustment problems similar to those faced by workers assigned to rotating shifts. Again, family and social responsibilities make it difficult for people to follow an exclusive night activity schedule. Workers with on-call schedules present a slightly different problem,

REFERENCES

1. Sack RL, Auckley D, Auger RR, et al. American Academy of Sleep Medicine. Circadian rhythm sleep disorders. Part I: basic principles, shift work and jet lag disorders. An American Academy of Sleep Medicine review. Sleep 2007; 30:1460–83.
2. Gonzalez MM, Aston-Jones G. Circadian regulation of arousal: role of the noradrenergic locus coeruleus system and light exposure. Sleep 2006; 29:1327–36.
3. Czeisler CA, Duffy JF, Shanahan TL, et al. Stability, precision, and near-24-hour period of the human circadian pacemaker. Science 1999; 284:2177–81.
4. Bartky IR, Dick SJ. The first time balls. J Hist Astronomy 1981; 12:155–64.
5. Zerubavel E. The standardization of time: a sociohistorical perspective. Am J Sociol 1982; 88:1–23.
6. Downing M. Spring Forward: The Annual Madness of Daylight Saving. Washington (DC): Shoemaker & Hoard, 2005.
7. Coren S. Daylight savings time and traffic accidents. N Engl J Med 1996; 334:924.
8. Toh KL, Jones CR, He Y, et al. An *hPer2* phosphorylation site mutation in familial advanced sleep phase syndrome. Science 2001; 291:1040–3.

9. Dagan Y, Eisenstein M. Circadian rhythm sleep disorders: toward a more precise definition and diagnosis. Chronobiol Int 1999;16: 213–22.

10. Sack RL, Lewy AJ, Blood ML, Keith LD, Nakagawa H. Circadian rhythm abnormalities in totally blind people: incidence and clinical significance. J Clin Endocrinol Metab 1992; 75:127–34.

11. Sack RL, Brandes RW, Kendall AR, Lewy AJ. Entrainment of free-running circadian rhythms by melatonin in blind people. N Engl J Med 2000; 343:1070–7.

12. Sack RL, Auckley D, Auger RR, et al; American Academy of Sleep Medicine. Circadian rhythm sleep disorders. Part II: advanced sleep phase disorder, delayed sleep phase disorder, free-running disorder, and irregular sleep-wake rhythm. An American Academy of Sleep Medicine review. Sleep 2007; 30:1484–501.

13. Leger D, Guilleminault C, Santos C, Paillard M. Sleep/wake cycles in the dark: sleep recorded by polysomnography in 26 totally blind subjects compared to controls. Clin Neurophysiol 2002; 113:1607–14.

14. Lewy AJ, Bauer VK, Hasler BP, Kendall AR, Pires ML, Sack RL. Capturing the circadian rhythms of free-running blind people with 0.5 mg melatonin. Brain Res 2001; 918:96–100.

15. Martin JL, Webber AP, Alam T, Harker JO, Josephson KR, Alessi CA. Daytime sleeping, sleep disturbance, and circadian rhythms in the nursing home. Am J Geriatr Psychiatry 2006; 14:121–9.

16. Foley D, Ancoli-Israel S, Britz P, Walsh J. Sleep disturbances and chronic disease in older adults: results of the 2003 National Sleep Foundation Sleep in America Survey. J Psychosom Res 2004; 56:497–502.

17. Schrader H, Bovim G, Sand T. The prevalence of delayed and advanced sleep phase syndromes. J Sleep Res 1993; 2:51–5.

18. Adan A, Natale V. Gender differences in morningness-eveningness preference. Chronobiol Int 2002; 19:709–20.

19. Ancoli-Israel S, Schnierow B, Kelsoe J, Fink R. A pedigree of one family with delayed sleep phase syndrome. Chronobiol Int 2001; 18:831–40.

20. Archer SN, Robilliard DL, Skene DJ, et al. A length polymorphism in the circadian clock gene Per3 is linked to delayed sleep phase syndrome and extreme diurnal preference. Sleep 2003; 26:413–5.

21. Pereira DS, Tufik S, Louzada FM, et al. Association of the length polymorphism in the human Per3 gene with the delayed sleep-phase syndrome: does latitude have an influence upon it? Sleep 2005; 28:29–32.

22. Iwase T, Kajimura N, Uchiyama M, et al. Mutation screening of the human CLOCK gene in circadian rhythm sleep disorders. Psychiatry Res 2002; 109:121–8.

23. Katzenberg D, Young T, Finn L, et al. A CLOCK polymorphism associated with human diurnal preference. Sleep 1998; 21:569–76.

24. Horne JA, Ostberg O. A self-assessment questionnaire to determine morningness-eveningness in human circadian rhythms. Int J Chronobiol 1976;4:97–110.

25. Dagan Y, Stein D, Steinbock M, Yovel I, Hallis D. Frequency of delayed sleep phase syndrome among hospitalized adolescent psychiatric patients. J Psychosom Res 1998; 45:15–20.

26. Morgenthaler TI, Lee-Chiong T, Alessi C, et al; Standards of Practice Committee of the American Academy of Sleep Medicine. Practice parameters for the clinical evaluation and treatment of circadian rhythm sleep disorders. An American Academy of Sleep Medicine report. Sleep 2007; 30:1445–59. Erratum in: Sleep 2008; 31.

27. Rosenthal NE, Joseph-Vanderpool JR, Levendosky AA, et al. Phase-shifting effects of bright morning light as treatment for delayed sleep phase syndrome. Sleep 1990; 13:354–61.

28. Krahn LE. Circadian Rhythm Disorders. In: Pagel JF, Pandi-Perumal SR, editors. Primary Care Sleep Medicine: A Practical Guide. Totowa (NJ): Humana Press, 2007. p. 261–74.

29. Arendt J, Deacon S, English J, Hampton S, Morgan L. Melatonin and adjustment to phase shift. J Sleep Res 1995; 4:74–9.

30. Kayumov L, Brown G, Jindal R, Buttoo K, Shapiro CM. A randomized, double-blind, placebo-controlled crossover study of the effect of exogenous melatonin on delayed sleep phase syndrome. Psychosom Med 2001; 63:40–8.

31. Nagtegaal JE, Kerkhof GA, Smits MG, Swart AC, Van Der Meer YG. Delayed sleep phase syndrome: a placebo-controlled cross-over study on the effects of melatonin administered five hours before the individual dim light melatonin onset. J Sleep Res 1998; 7:135–43.

32. Lu BS, Zee PC. Circadian rhythm sleep disorders. Chest 2006; 130:1915–23.

33. Ito A, Ando K, Hayakawa T, et al. Long-term course of adult patients with delayed sleep phase syndrome. Jpn J Psychiatry Neurol 1993; 47:563–7.

34. Campbell SS, Dawson D, Anderson MW. Alleviation of sleep maintenance insomnia with timed exposure to bright light. J Am Geriatr Soc 1993; 41:829–36.

35. Murphy PJ, Campbell SS. Enhanced performance in elderly subjects following bright light treatment of sleep maintenance insomnia. J Sleep Res 1996; 5:165–72.

36. De Leersnyder H, Bresson JL, de Blois MC, et al. Beta 1-adrenergic antagonists and melatonin reset the clock and restore sleep in a circadian disorder, Smith-Magenis syndrome. J Med Genet 2003; 40:74–8.

37. Sack RL. Clinical practice: jet lag. N Engl J Med 2010; 4:440–7.

38. Petrie K, Dawson AG, Thompson L, Brook R. A double-blind trial of melatonin as a treatment for jet lag in international cabin crew. Biol Psychiatry 1993; 33:526–30.

39. Spitzer RL, Terman M, Williams JB, et al. Jet lag: clinical features, validation of a new syndrome-specific scale, and lack of response to melatonin in a randomized, double-blind trial. Am J Psychiatry 1999; 156:1392–6.

40. Wright SW, Lawrence LM, Wrenn KD, Haynes ML, Welch LW, Schlack HM. Randomized clinical trial of melatonin after night-shift work: efficacy and neuropsychologic effects. Ann Emerg Med 1998; 32:334–40.

41. Mohren DC, Jansen NW, Kant IJ, Galama J, van den Brandt PA, Swaen GM. Prevalence of common infections among employees in different work schedules. J Occup Environ Med 2002; 44:1003–11. Erratum in: J Occup Environ Med 2003; 45: 105.

42. Czeisler CA, Moore-Ede MC, Coleman RH. Rotating shift work schedules that disrupt sleep are improved by applying circadian principles. Science 1982; 217:460–3.

43. Rosekind MR, Smith RM, Miller DL, et al. Alertness management: strategic naps in operational settings. J Sleep Res 1995; 4:62–6.

44. Hart CL, Ward AS, Haney M, Foltin RW. Zolpidem-related effects on performance and mood during simulated night-shift work. Exp Clin Psychopharmacol 2003;11:259–68.

45. Nickelsen T, Samel A, Vejvoda M, Wenzel J, Smith B, Gerzer R. Chronobiotic effects of the melatonin agonist LY 156735 following a simulated 9h time shift: results of a placebo-controlled trial. Chronobiol Int 2002; 19:915–36.